The LAB Project and Healthy Tales Production Present:

# Liza and Bert's Health Adventures!

## Volume 4: Bert's Picky Pizza

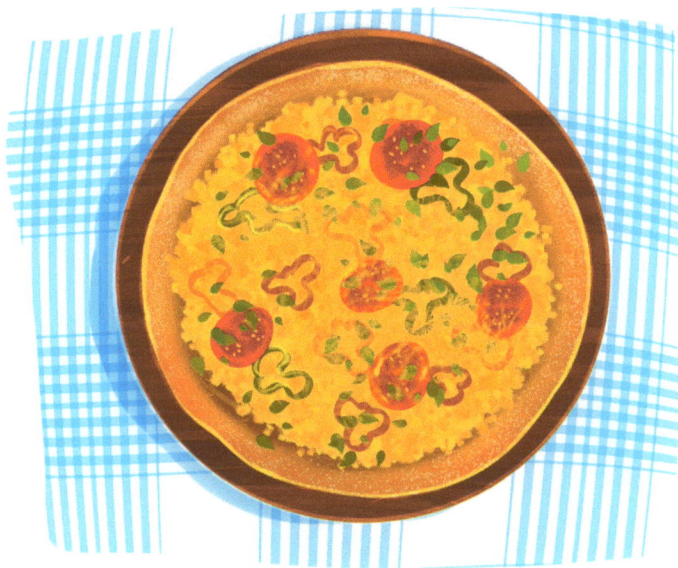

written by:
Aimee Curley, RN, MSN
Raphael L. Aquino, MHCI

illustrated by:
Ilhama Hamidova

# Dedication

To Zowee and Lauren, thank you for eating your vegetables as kids and inspiring me to write this book.

To Anna, thank you for being my number one fan.

To Nanay, I hope I make you proud.

-Raphael


This book is dedicated to my boys, Jack and Davis, and to my husband Tim and to my mom, Thelma, who always made sure I ate my veggies.

-Aimee

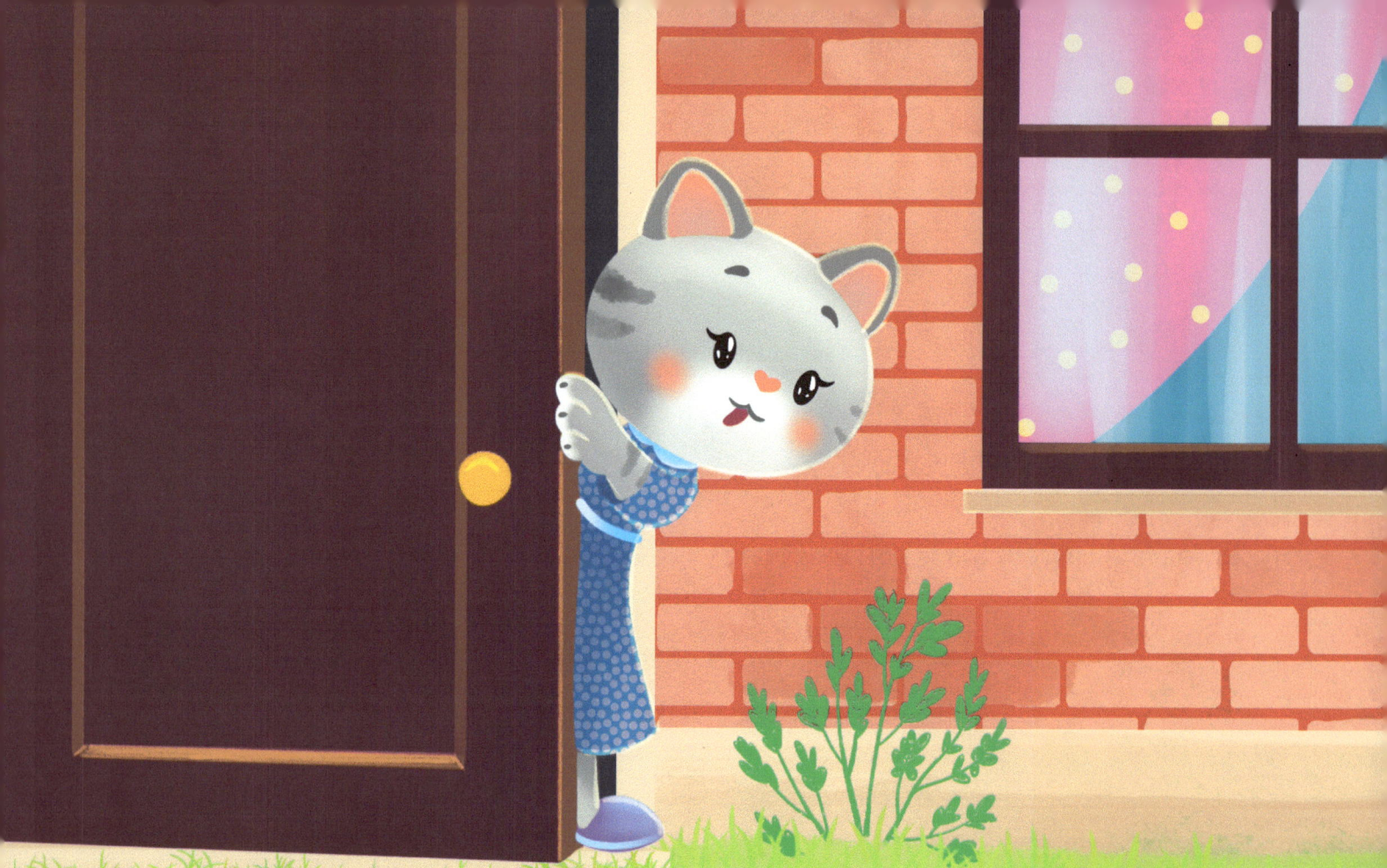

Liza the Lion and Bert the Bear are outside playing when Aunt Cathy the Cat calls, "Hey guys, come on inside. It's time to get ready for dinner!"

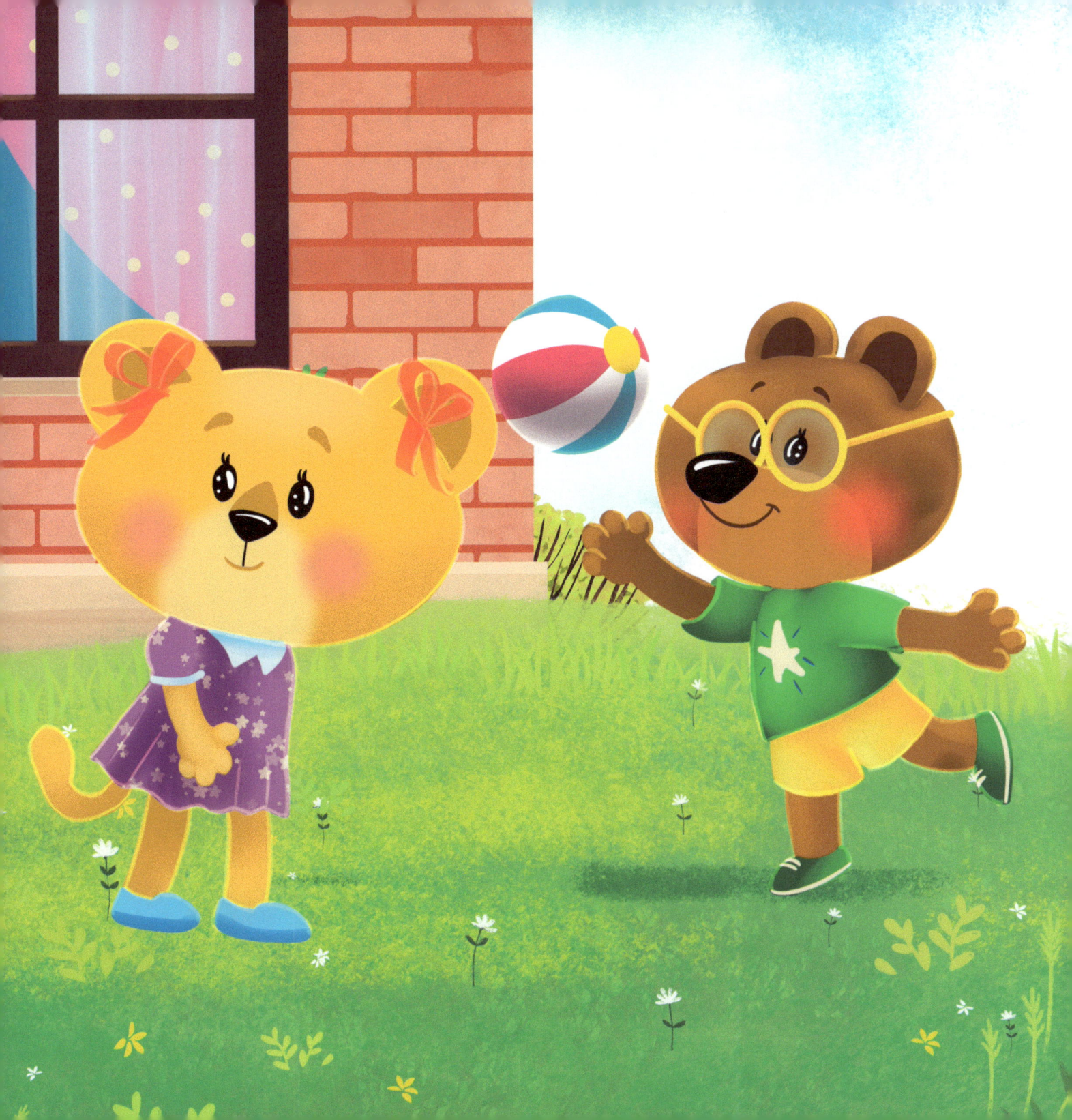

Bert and Liza run to the house, wash their hands, and take their seats at the table. "I'm so hungry! What are we having for dinner, Aunt Cathy?" asks Liza.

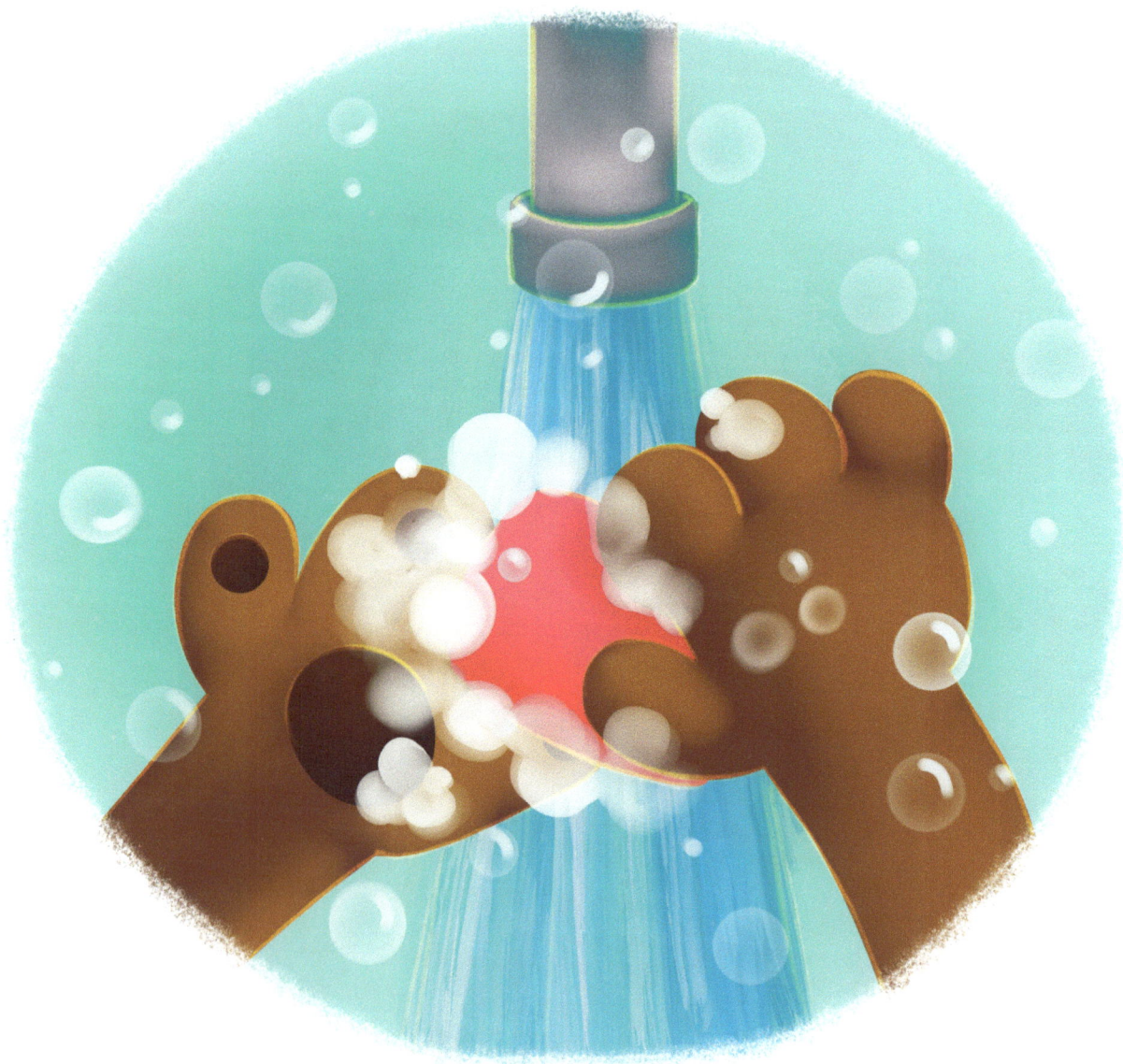

Aunt Cathy places a plate of grilled chicken and vegetables on the table. "Mmmm, it all smells so yummy!" says Liza.

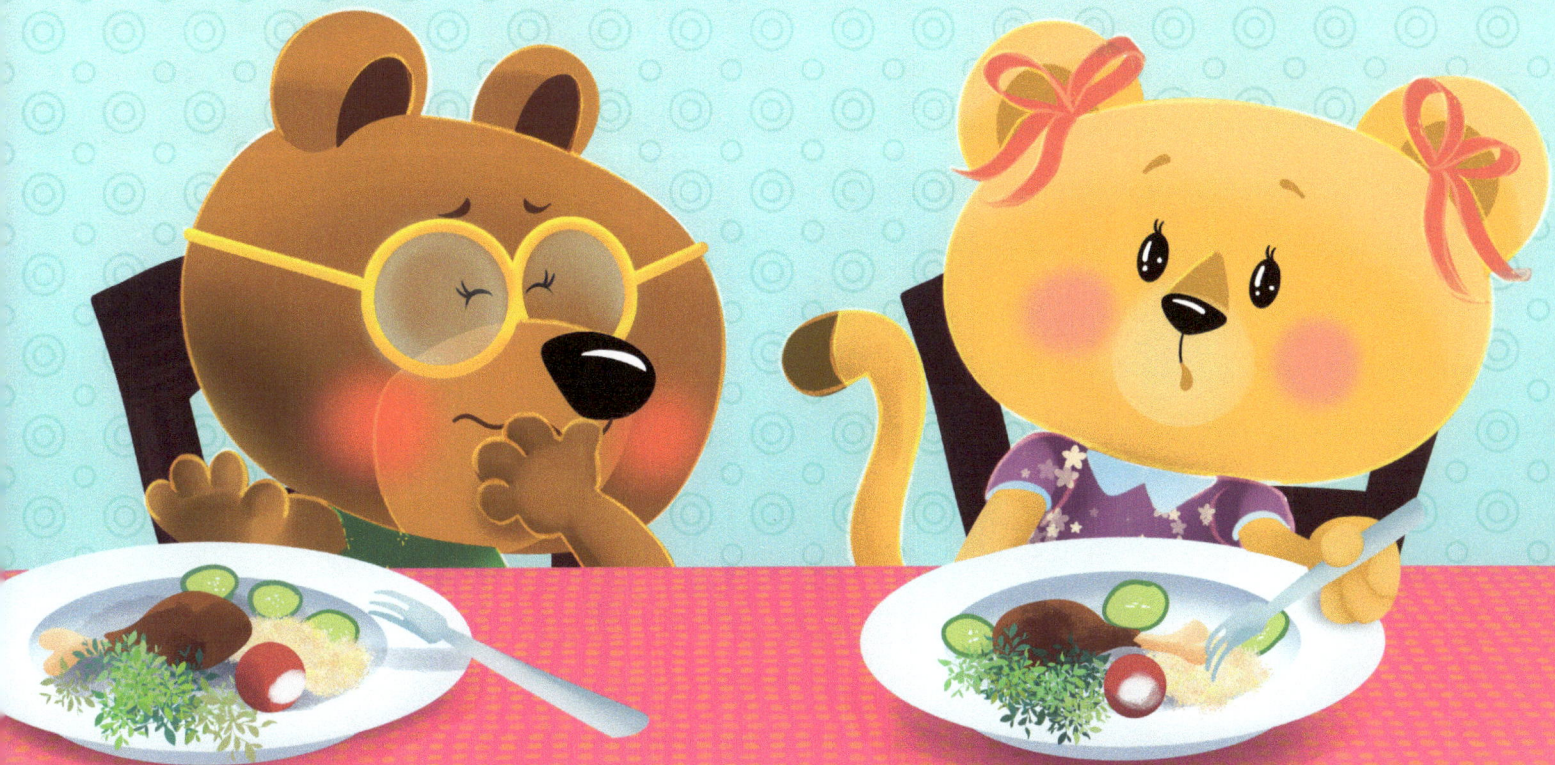

Bert sinks back in his chair, pushing his plate away from him.

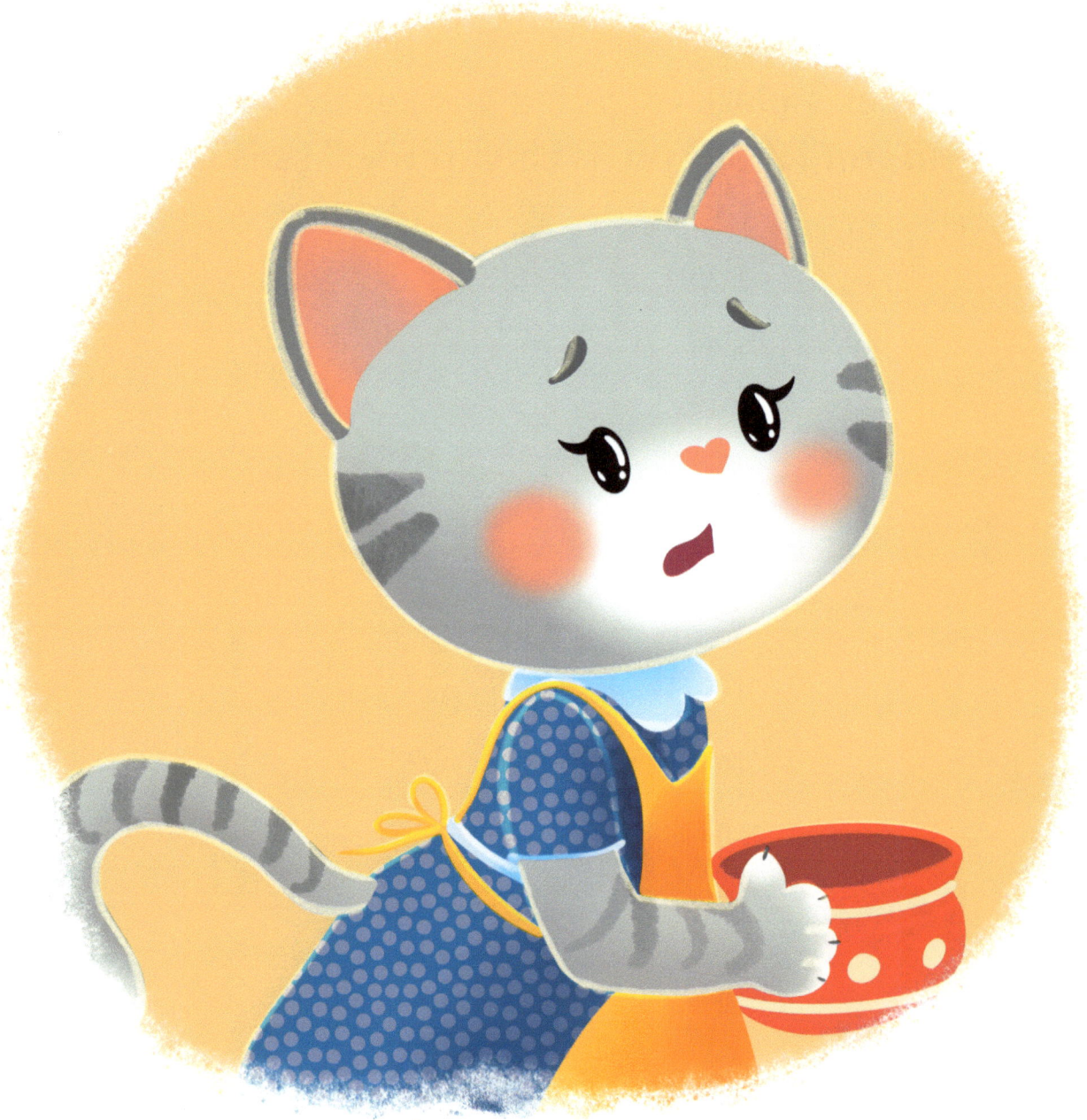

"What's the matter, Bert?" Aunt Cathy asks, "Aren't you hungry?"

"I was." says Bert, "but I just don't think I like chicken, and I do NOT want any of those vegetables. YUCK!"

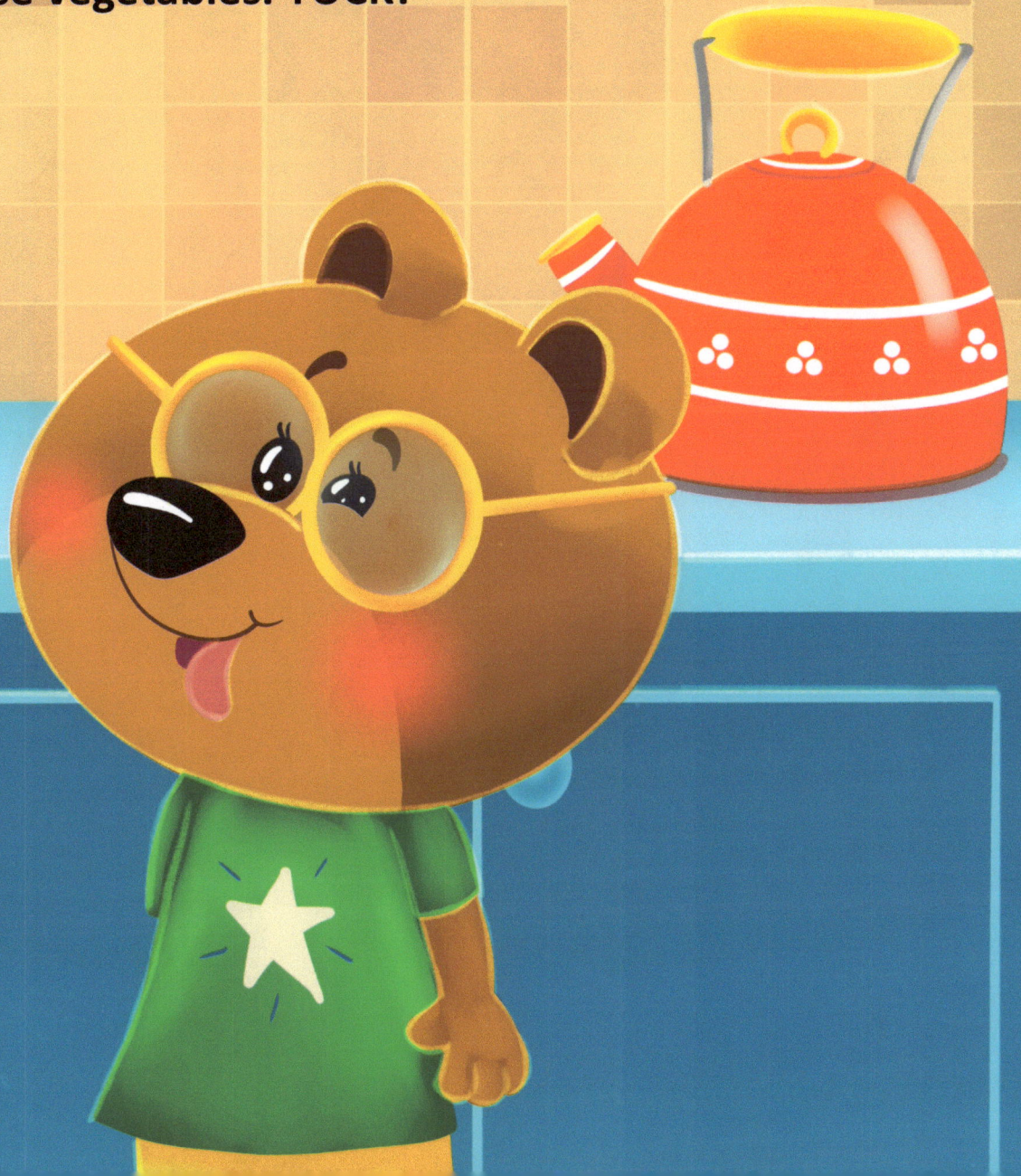

Aunt Cathy says, "But Bert, you said you loved this dish when I made it last week."

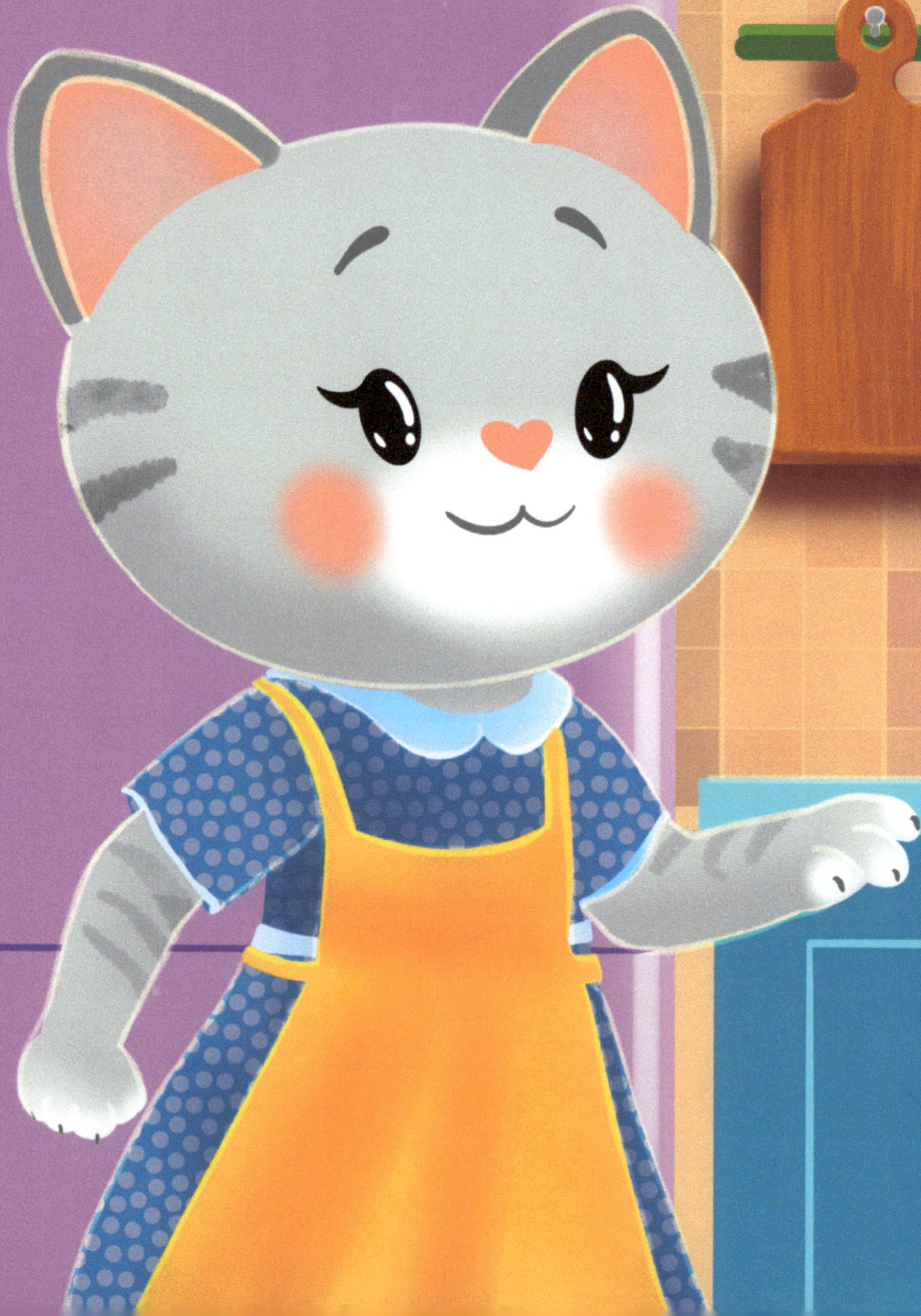

"Well, I don't like chicken anymore. . . and I really only like carrots now," Bert replies.

"YAY! More dinner for me!" Liza exclaims as she gobbles down another bite.

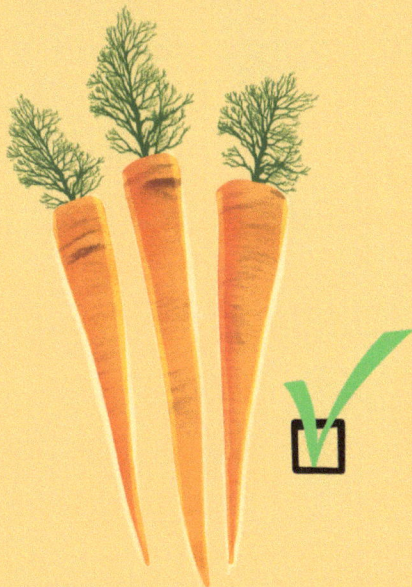

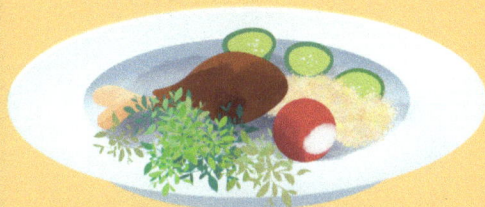

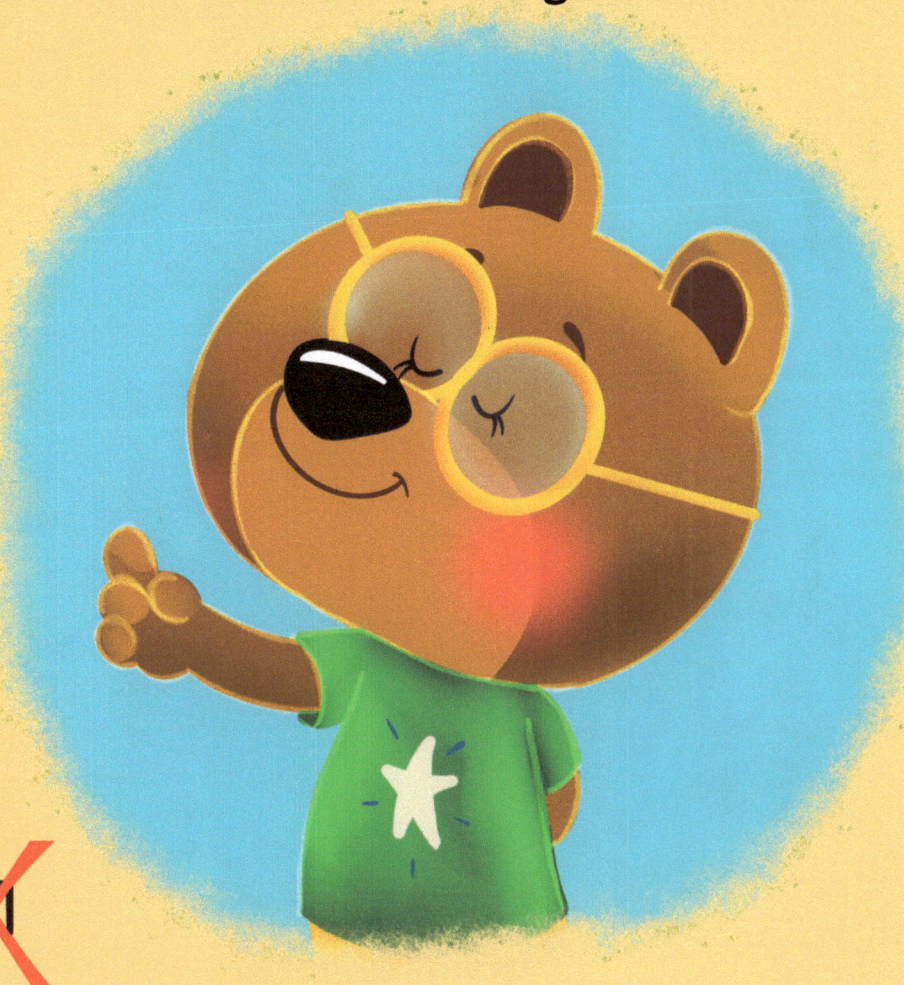

Bert asks if he could have last night's leftovers instead. Aunt Cathy agrees, and Bert takes out last night's leftover chili.

"Aunt Cathy, do you think I can make a different sandwich for lunch tomorrow?" asks Bert. "I don't want peanut butter and jelly."

"No peanut butter and Jelly, Bert?" questions Liza, "but that's your favorite!"

"Not anymore," says Bert. "Peanut butter is yucky!"

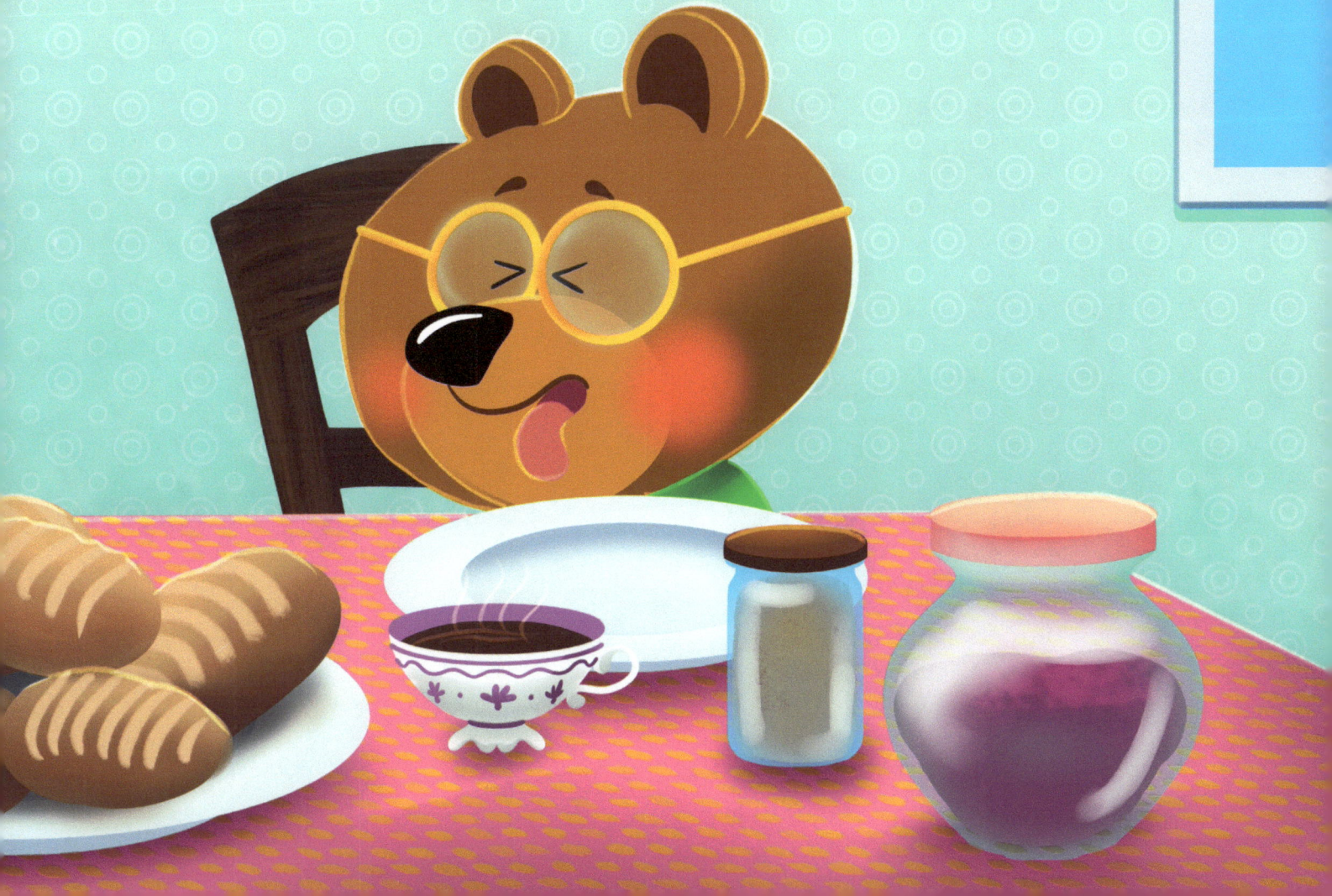

The next day, Aunt Cathy asks Bert and Liza if they want to go to the grocery store with her. "I think it would be good to plan for some lunches and dinners that we all enjoy," Aunt Cathy says.

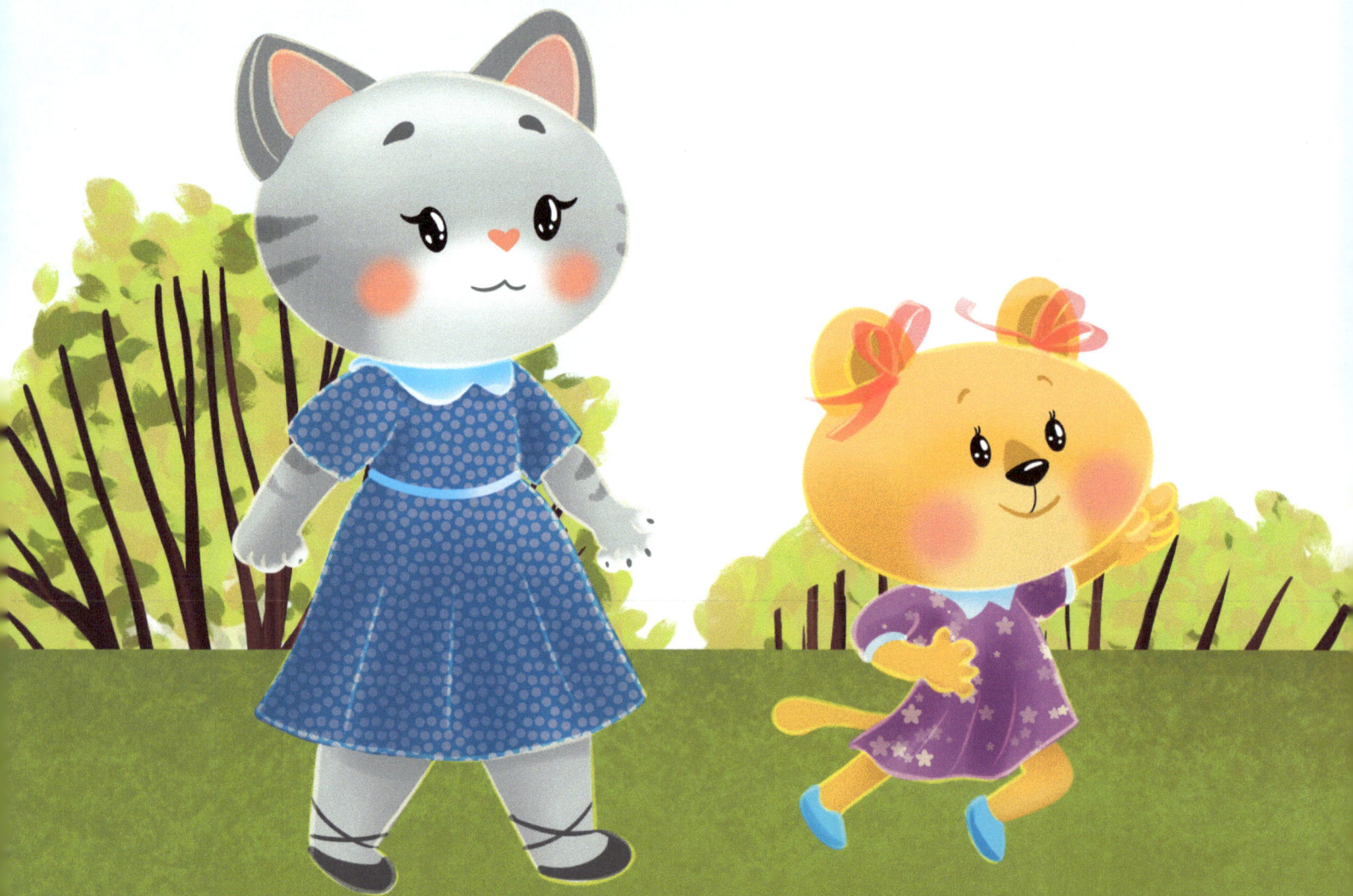

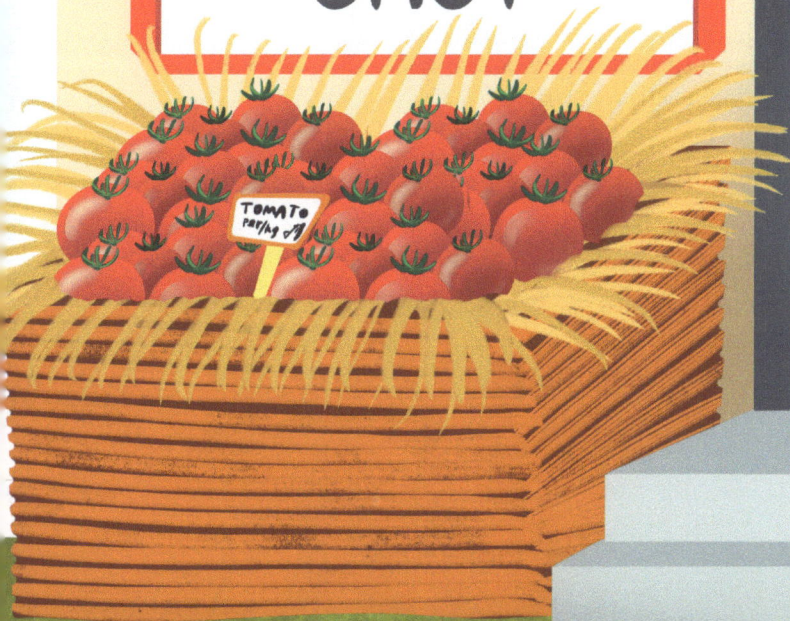

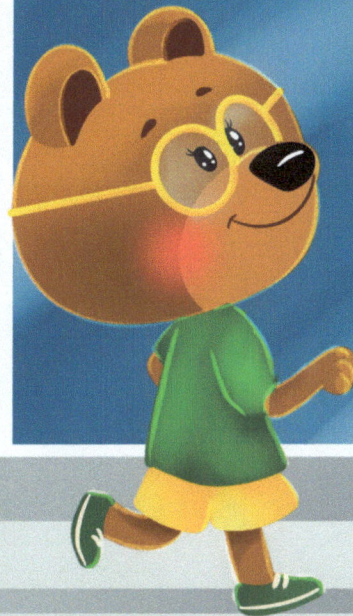

Bert and Liza agree that it would be fun to help with grocery shopping and pick out some foods that they like!

Aunt Cathy, Liza, and Bert drive over to the market. Once inside, Bert runs to the candy aisle and laughs "Ooohhh, I chose gummy bears!"

"Gummy bears?" Aunt Cathy asks. "Silly bear, you can't have candy for your lunch and dinner choices. Let's go to the produce, and you may each choose one fruit and vegetable you want to try".

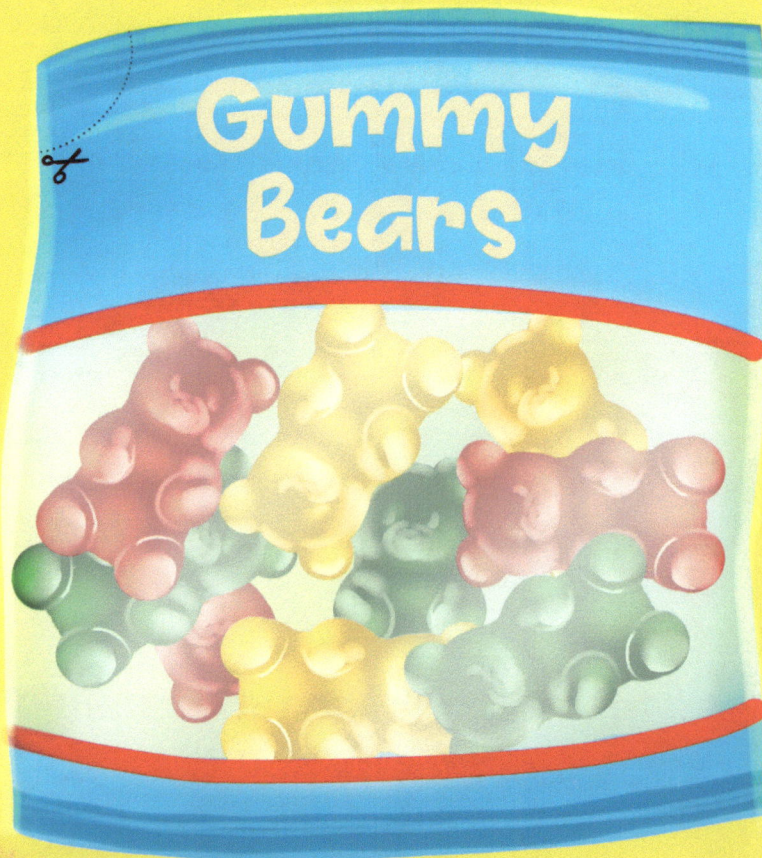

Once at the produce department, Liza quickly picks up a container of blueberries and a head of cauliflower.

 "I LOVE blueberries, and my friend, Davis the Duck, made tacos with crispy cauliflower the other day, and it was DELICIOUS!  Maybe we can get the recipe from his mom!" says Liza.

"What a wonderful idea!" cheers Aunt Cathy.

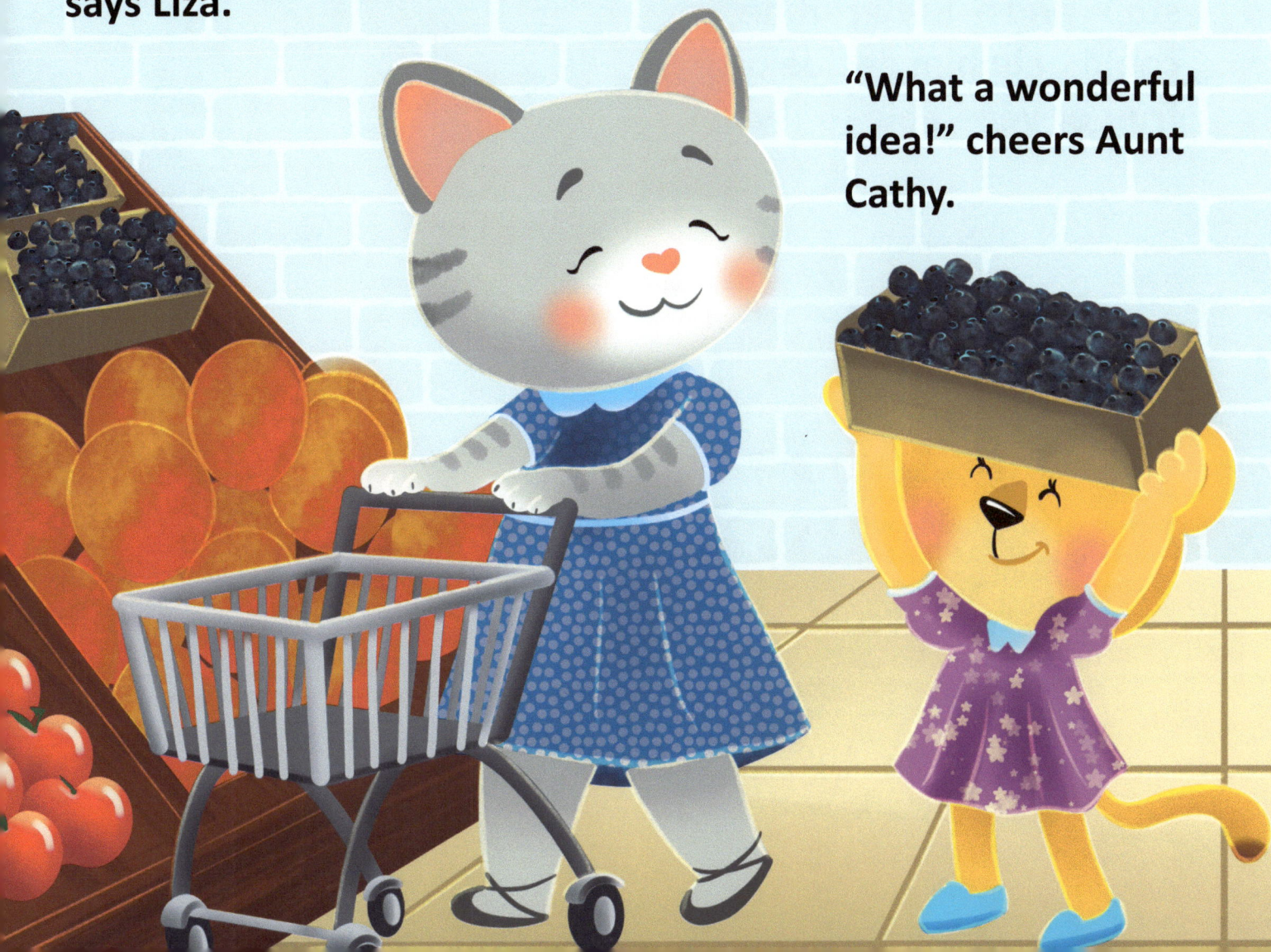

Meanwhile, Bert is having trouble finding a fruit or vegetable he wants to try. Suddenly, Jack the Jack Rabbit, the market manager, stops and asks Bert if he could help him decide on a fruit or vegetable to try.

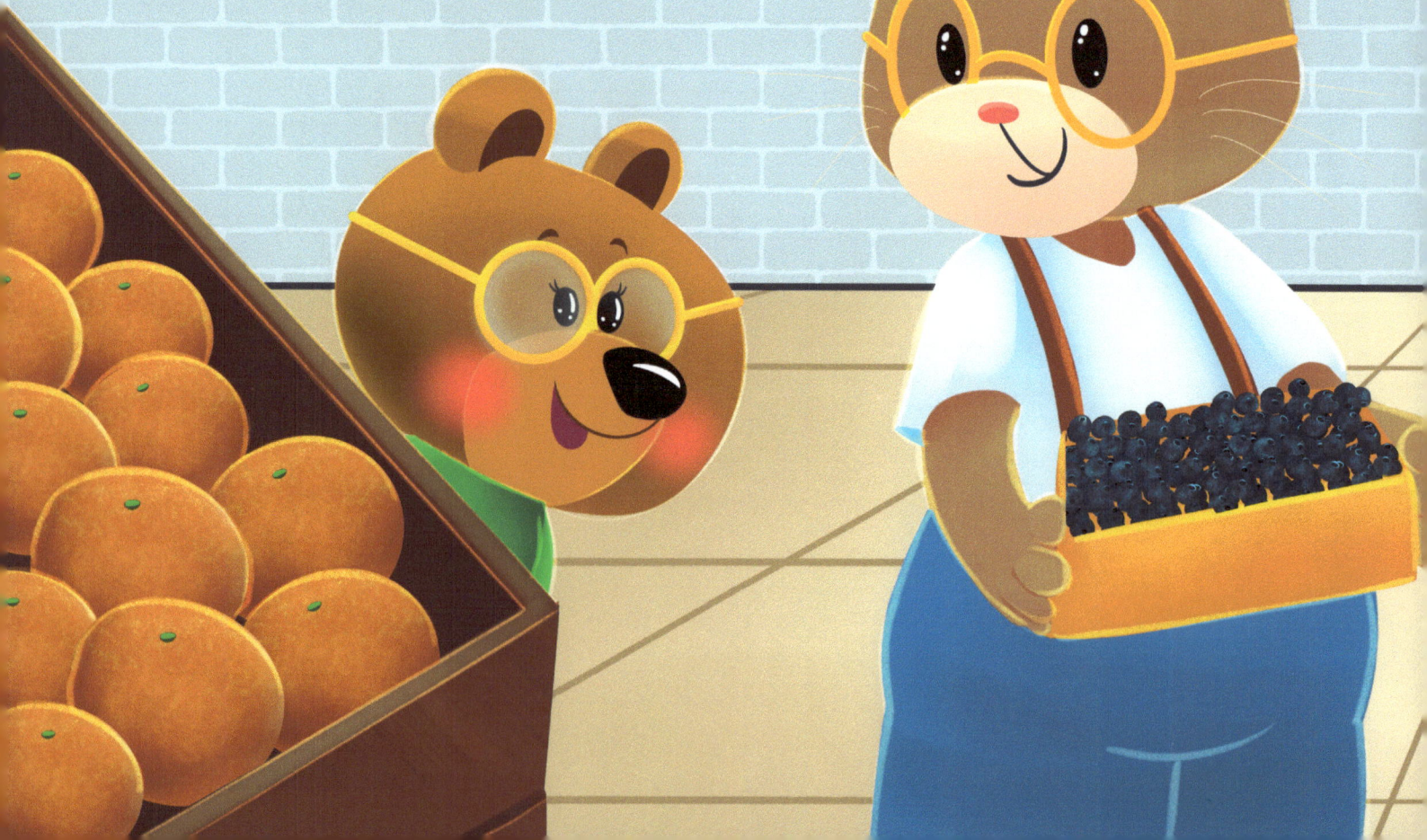

"What is your favorite food, Bert?" Jack asks.

"Pizza. I LOVE pizza!" Bert replies.

"Perfect!" says Jack. "Let's find something you may want to try on a pizza!" Jack says as he walks him over to the red peppers.

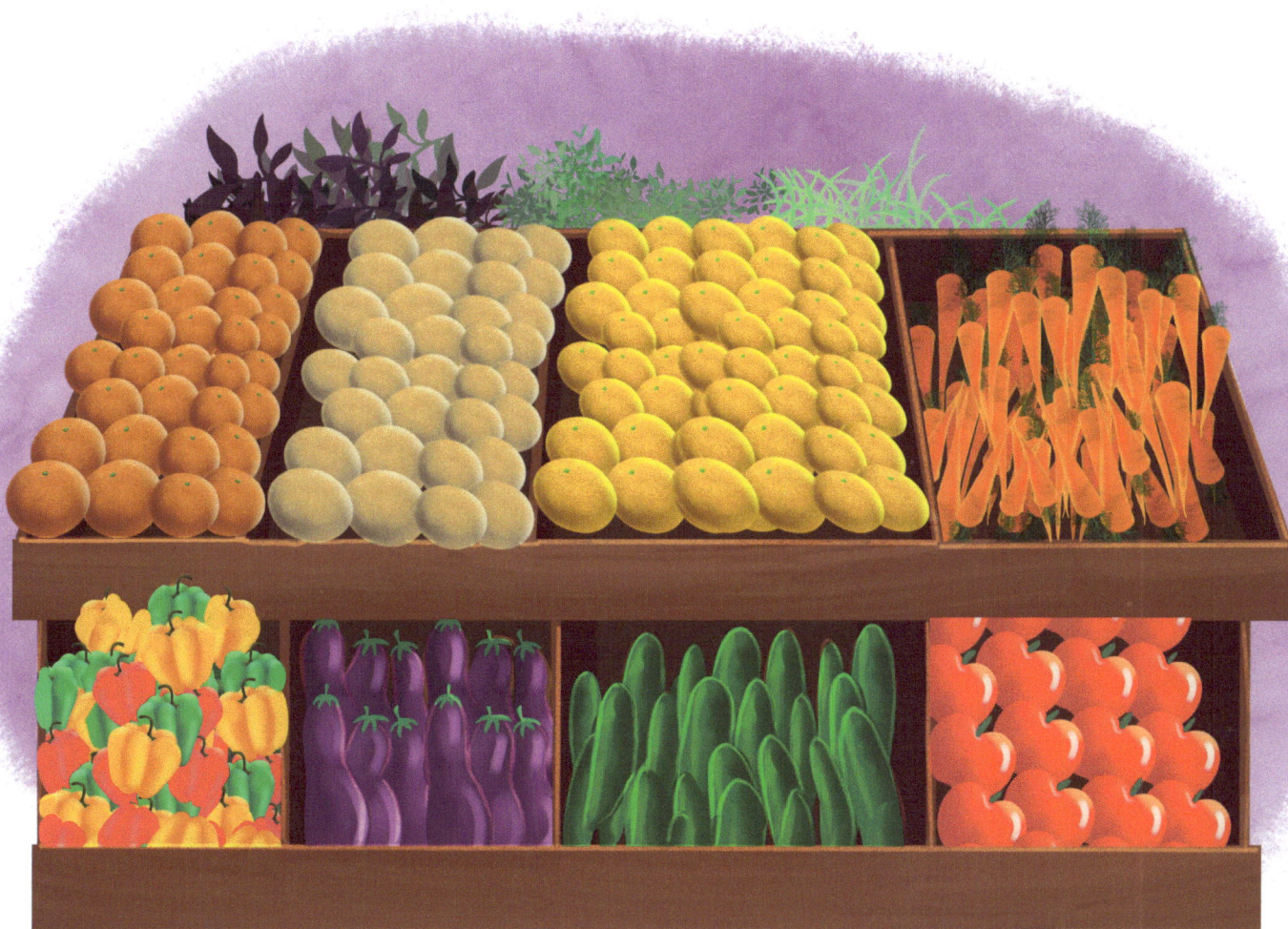

"What about this?" Jack says, holding up a red bell pepper. "Peppers have a nice crunch to them and just a little bit of sweetness."

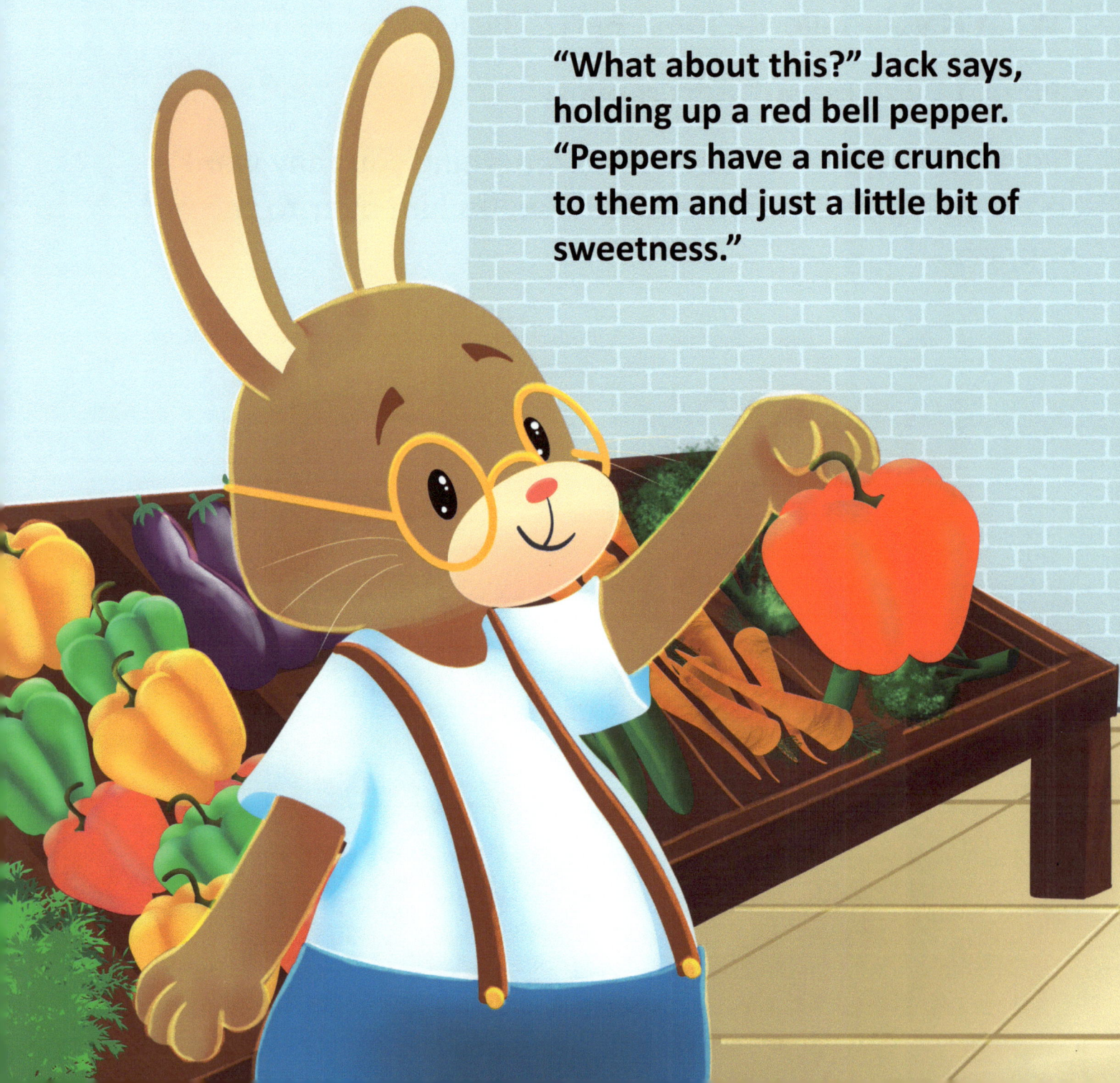

"A PEPPER? I'm not too sure about a pepper!" Bert says.

Jack laughs, "Well, you won't know until you try it! . . . And if you don't like it, you can come back and try something else until you find a pizza topping you like!"

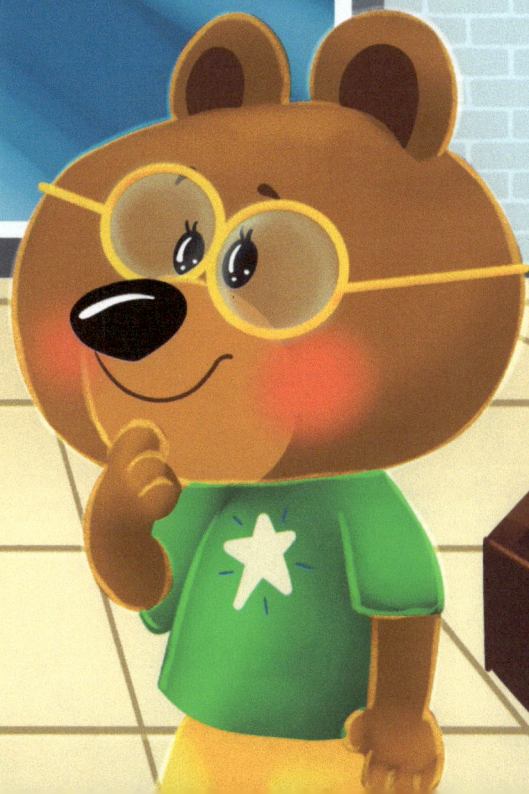

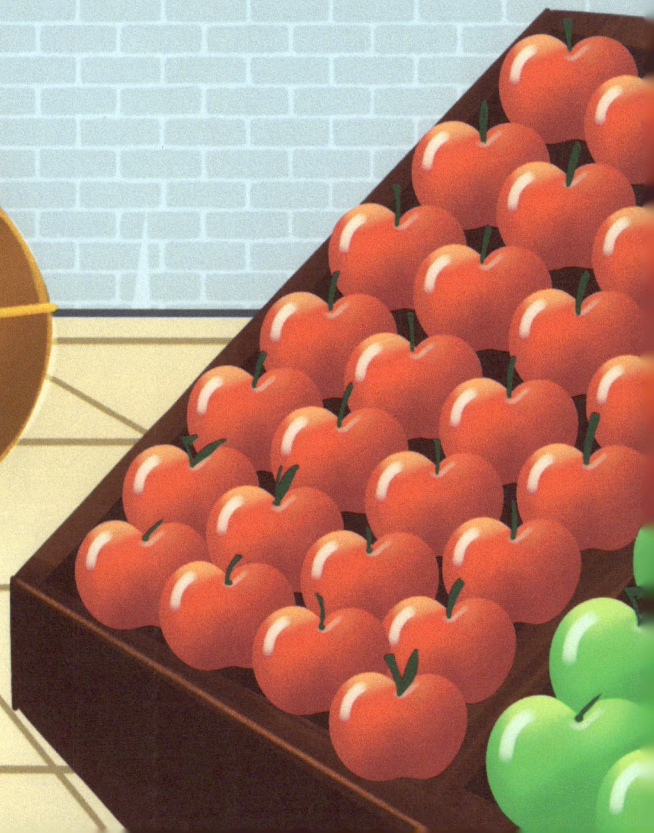

"Sometimes when you try things, you find out you don't like them. . . . but sometimes when you try things, you find out that you DO!" Aunt Cathy says.

"So if I try it and don't like it, I don't have to eat all of it, right?" asks Bert.

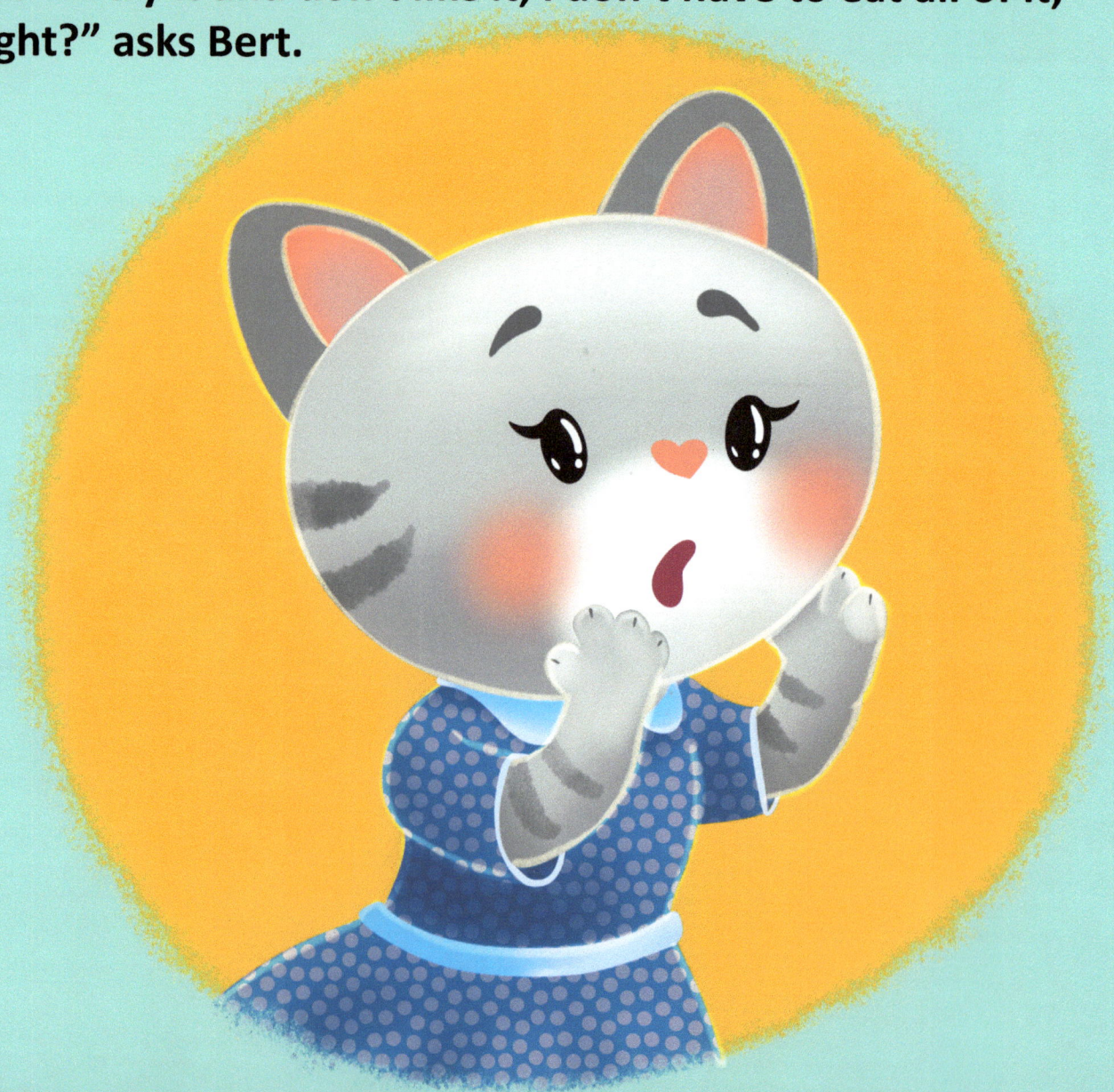

"That's right, Bert," Aunt Cathy assures him. "Sometimes, you have to try foods more than once before deciding whether you like them or not...

and sometimes, you have to try a food you don't like in a different way, like . . ."

"ON A PIZZA!" Bert, Liza, and Jack the Grocer all say together.

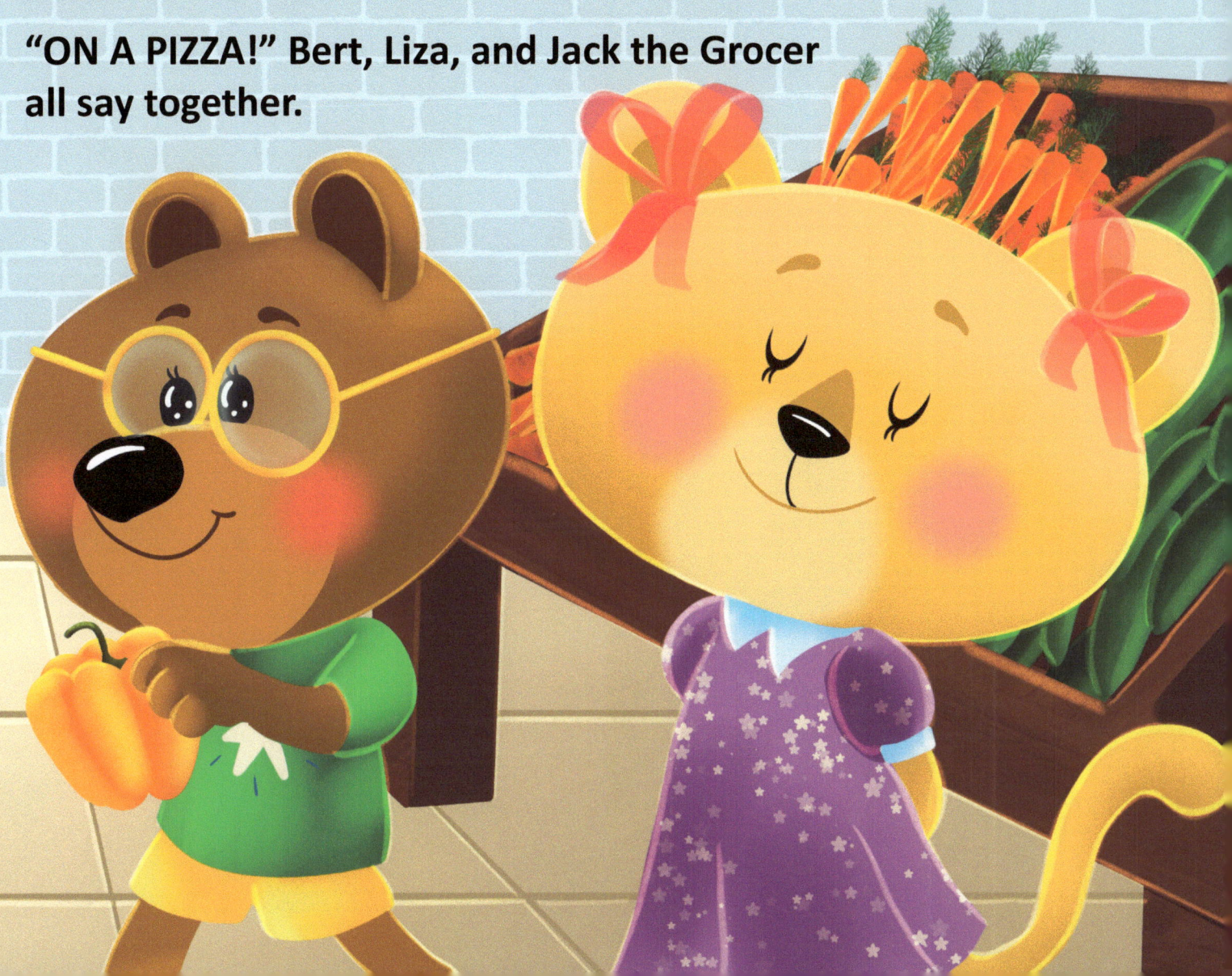

Bert took the red pepper, grabbed a few green apples, thanked Jack, and went to the check-out line.

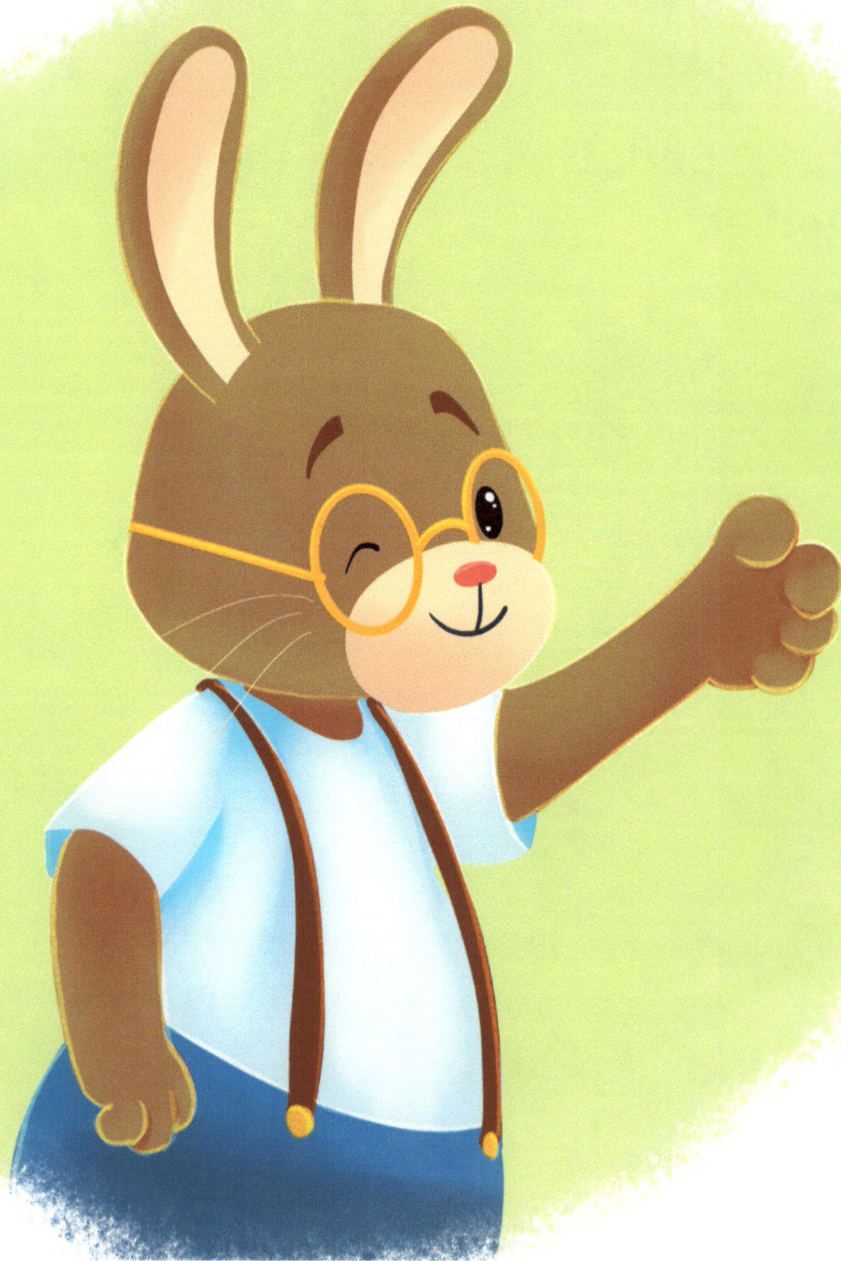

Make sure you let me know how your pizza turns out, Bert!"
Jack calls out.

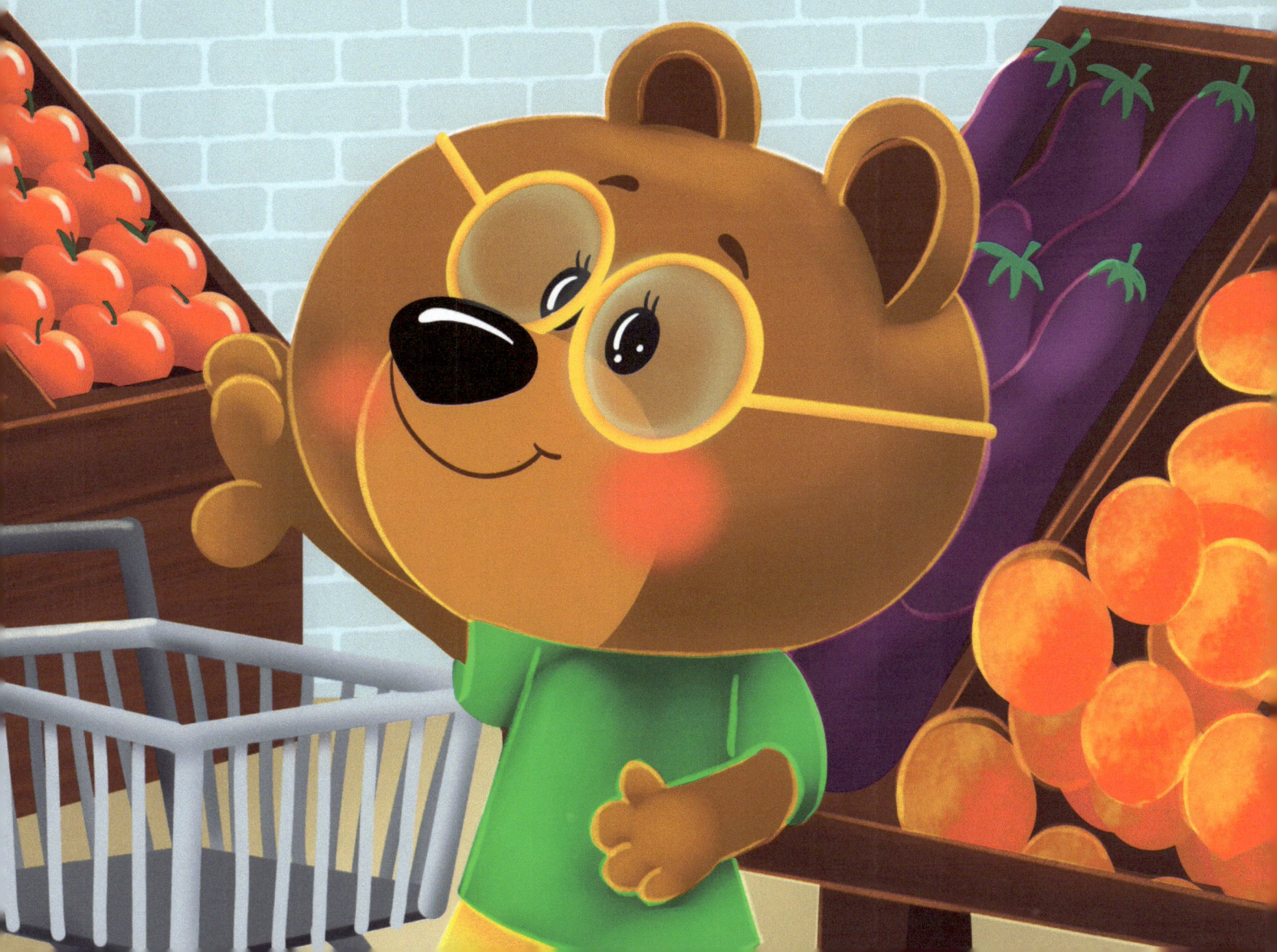

Once they returned to the house, Bert and Liza help Aunt Cathy bring the groceries inside.

"Can we make my special pizza tonight?" Bert asks.

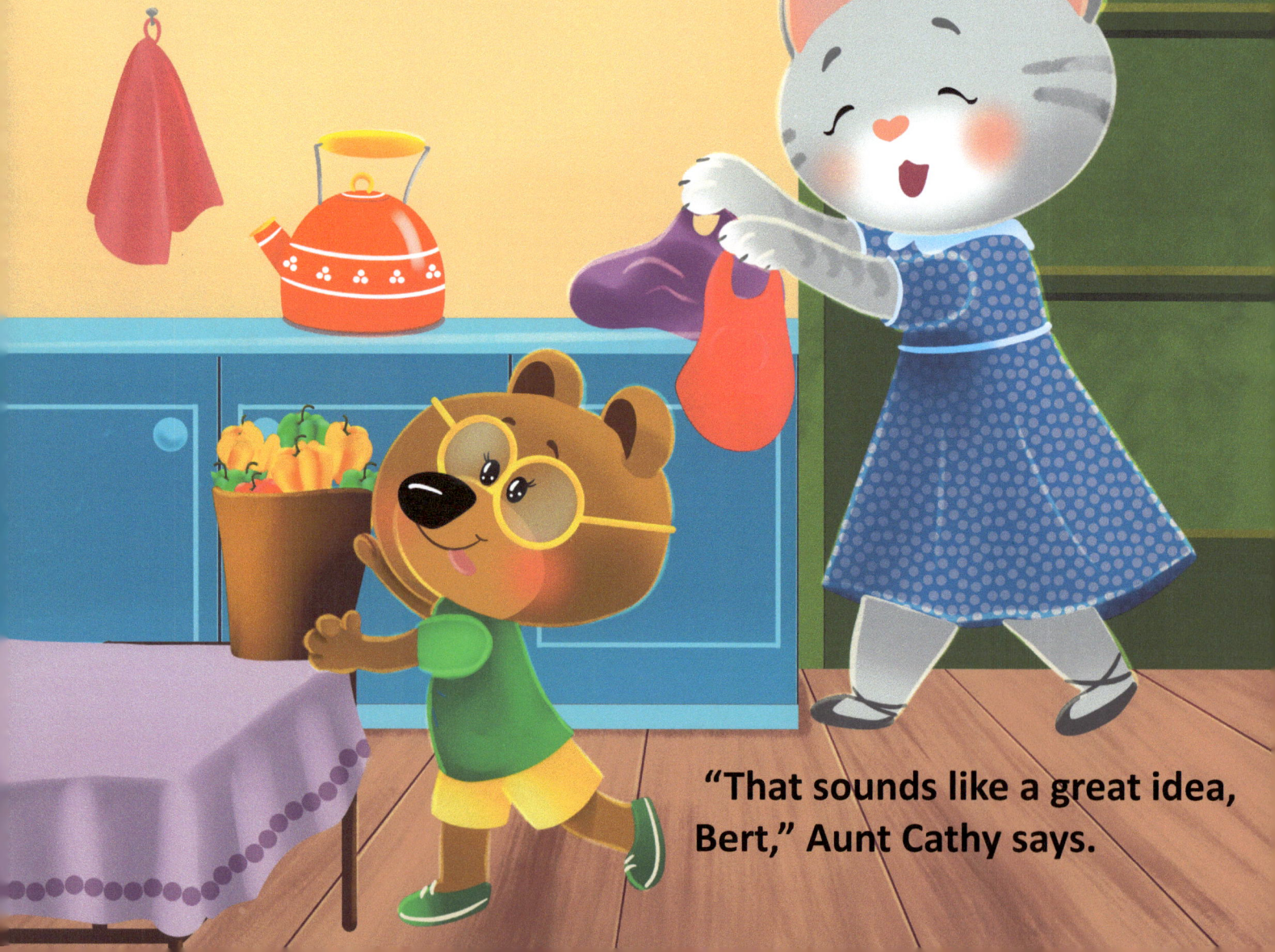

"That sounds like a great idea, Bert," Aunt Cathy says.

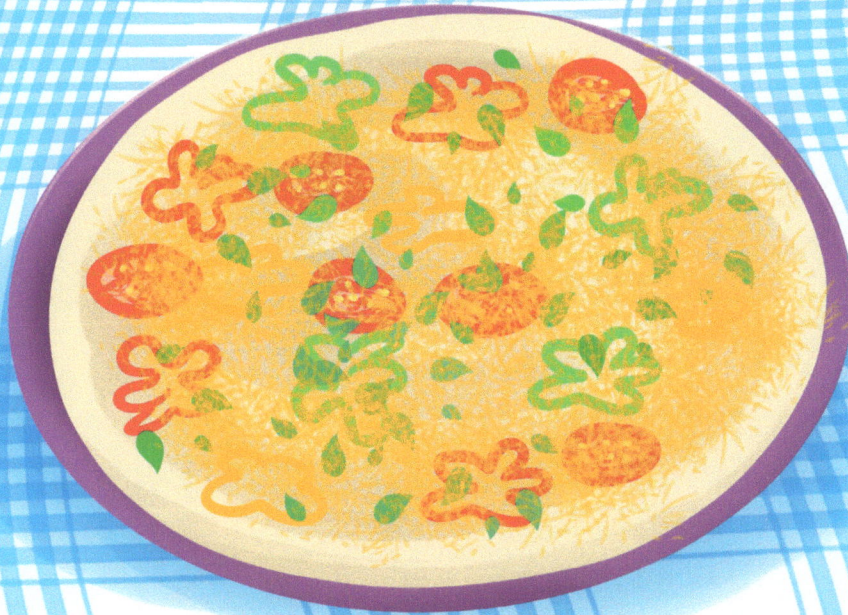

They all take turns washing their hands and getting the ingredients to make Bert's special pizza.

They roll the dough, add a little fresh tomato sauce, and slice the red pepper.

Bert, Liza, and Aunt Cathy add some shredded cheese and sliced red peppers to Bert's pizza, and soon, it is ready to go into the oven!

Bert and Liza sit in front of the oven, looking at the pizza. The room fills with the delicious smell of pizza.

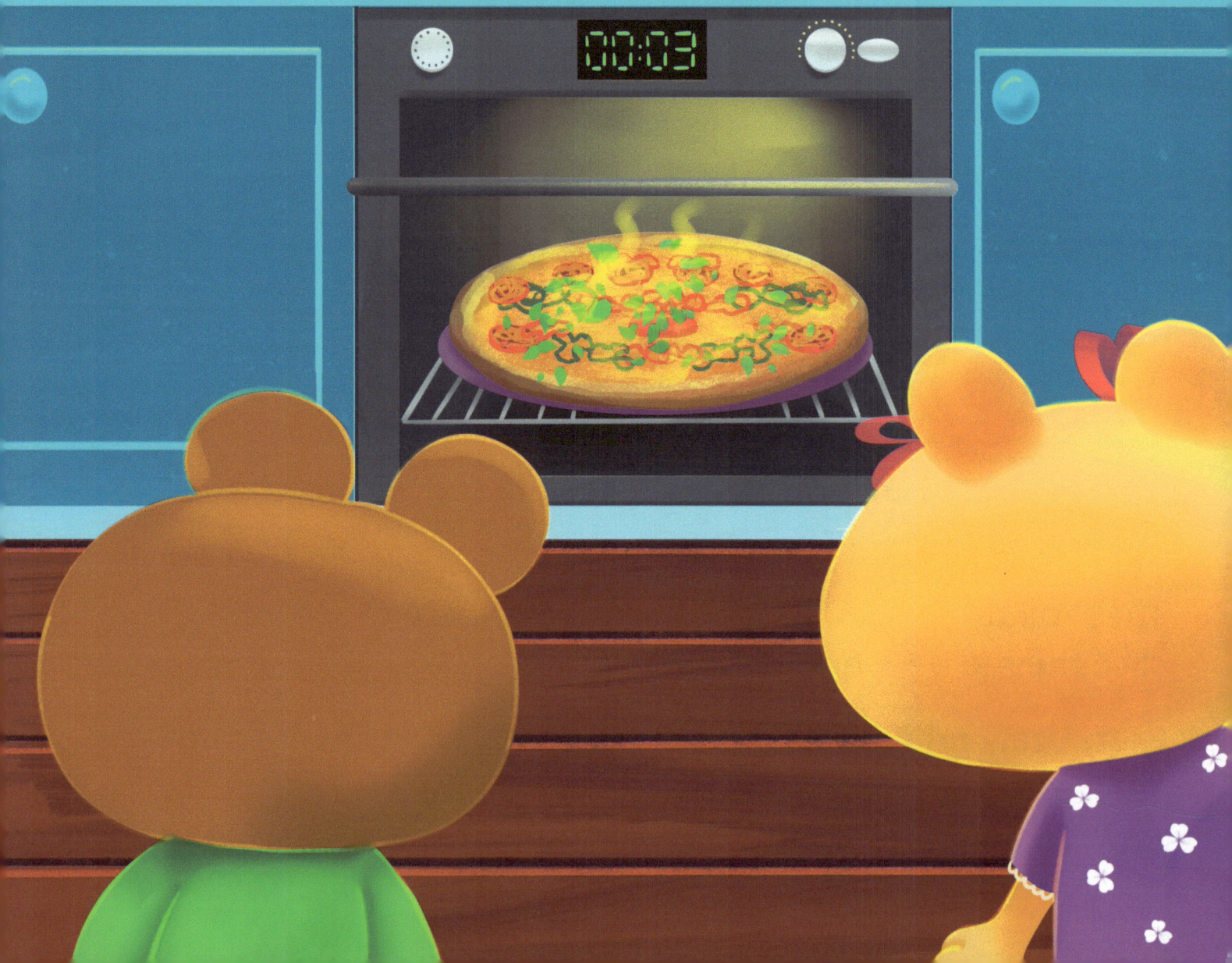

"Ohhhh, I see the cheese melting and bubbling," says Bert. "Do you think it is ready yet?"

"Just a few more minutes, and we can take it out and let it cool down," says Aunt Cathy.

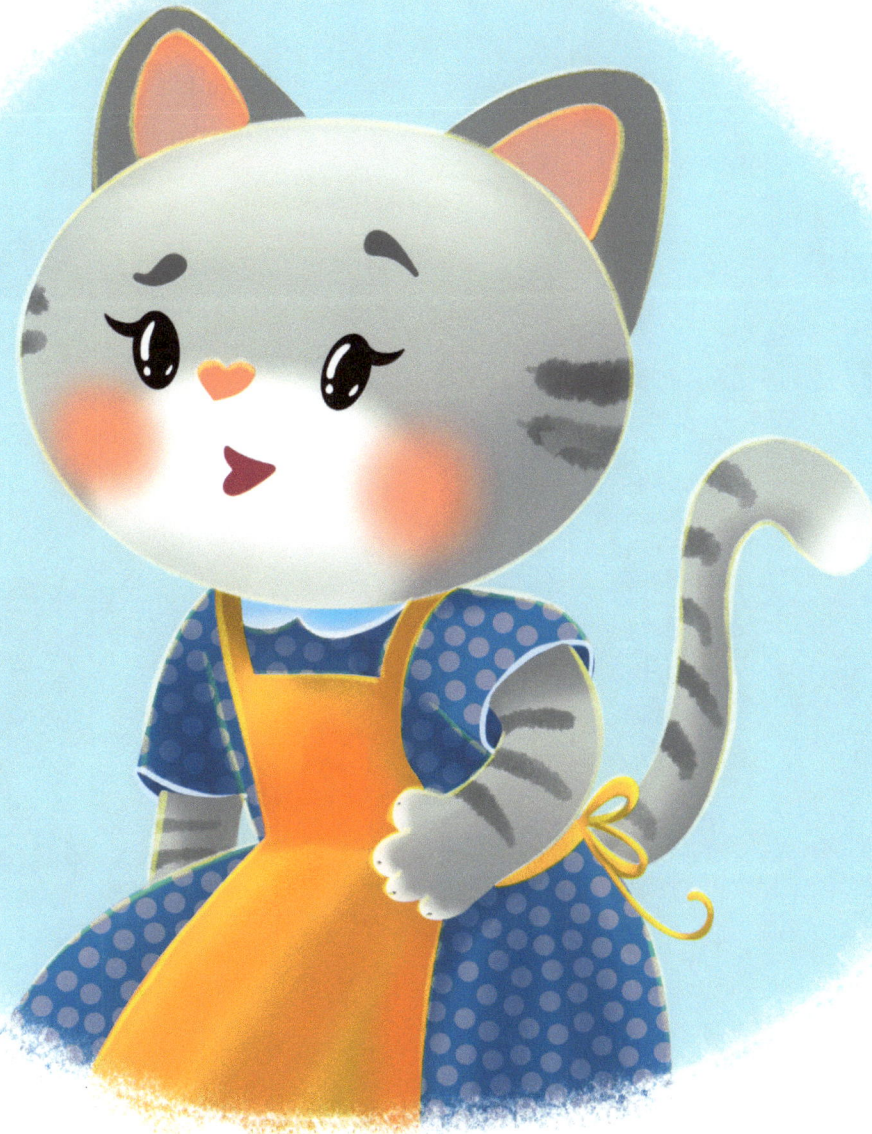

Not too long after, the pizza comes out of the oven and cool enough to try.

"Bert MUST have the first piece," says Liza. "After all, this is his special pizza."

Aunt Cathy puts a slice of the red pepper pizza on Bert's plate.

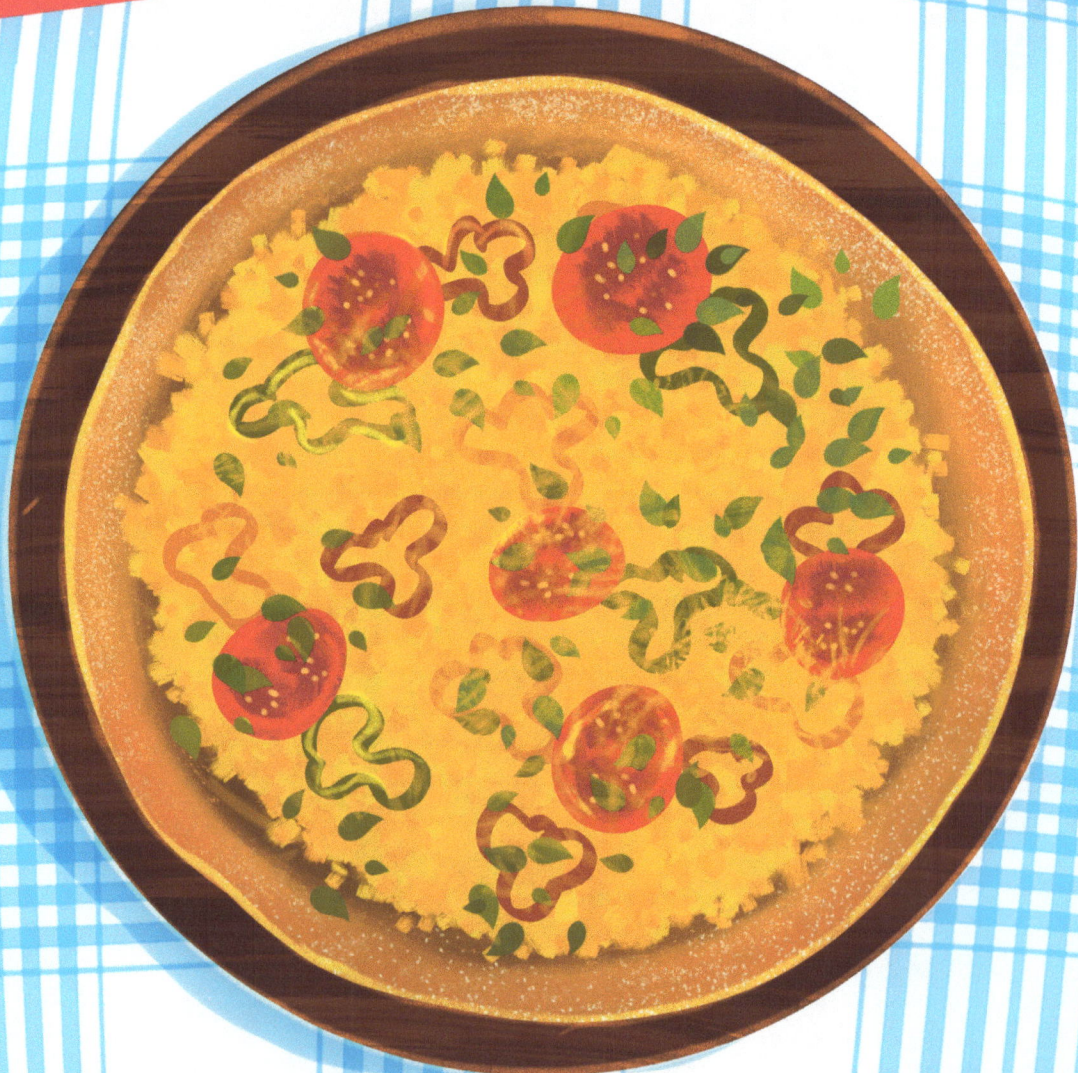

Bert looks at the slice, holds it up, looks over and under it, and turns it side to side. He smells it. "It smells good!"

Lisa said, "Oh, Bert, will you just take your bite? I'm hungry!" They all laugh . . .

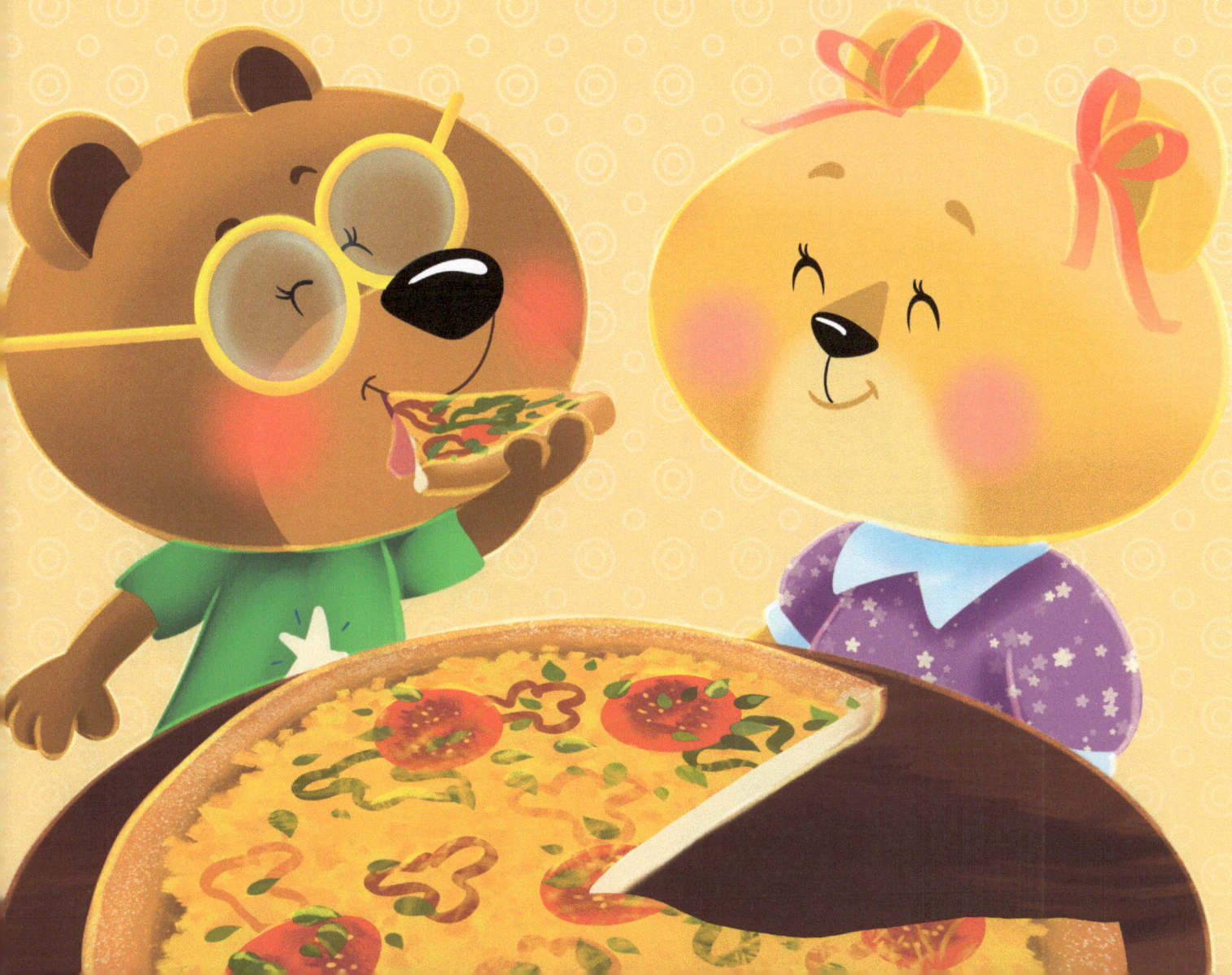

... and Bert takes a big bite of his pizza . . . red peppers and all.

Liza and Aunt Cathy wait for his reaction. . .

A big smile comes across Bert's face as he takes another big bite.

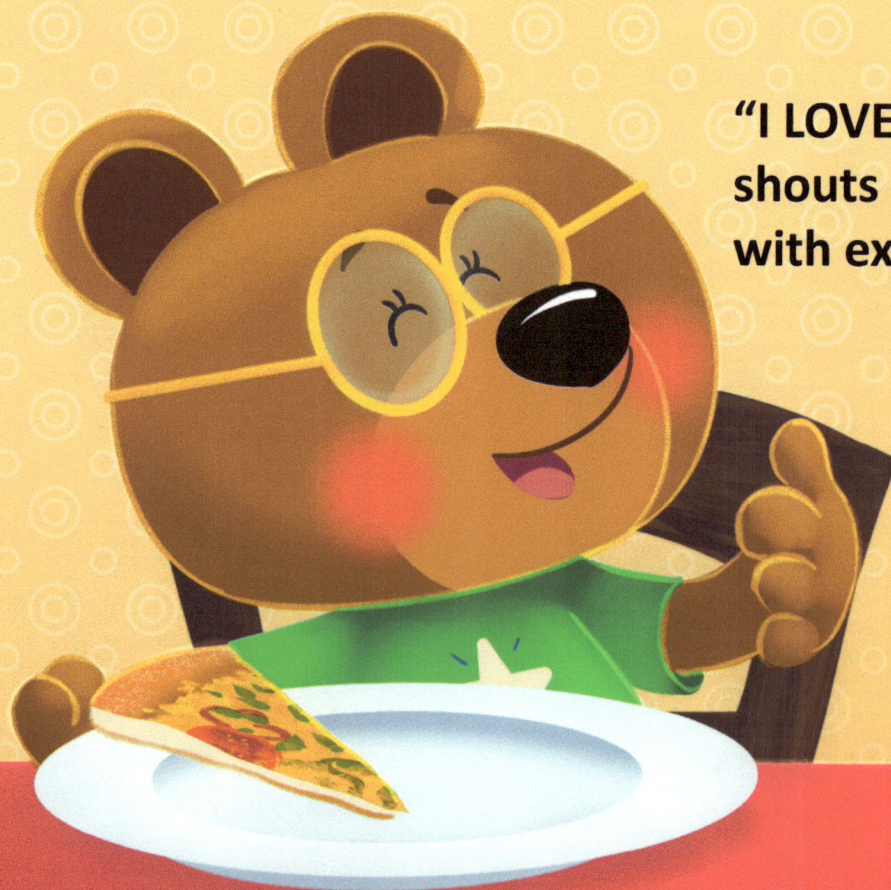

"I LOVE IT!" shouts Bert with excitement.

"I really like the way the red peppers crunch and taste a little sweet, and they mix well with the melty cheese and . . ."

"Okay, okay, Bert," Liza interrupts. "I'm hungry, and I want to try a piece!" They all laugh as Aunt Cathy serves up the pizza. They all agree that they enjoy the red peppers on the pizza, and Bert cannot wait to tell Jack the Jack Rabbit about his successful new pizza topping!

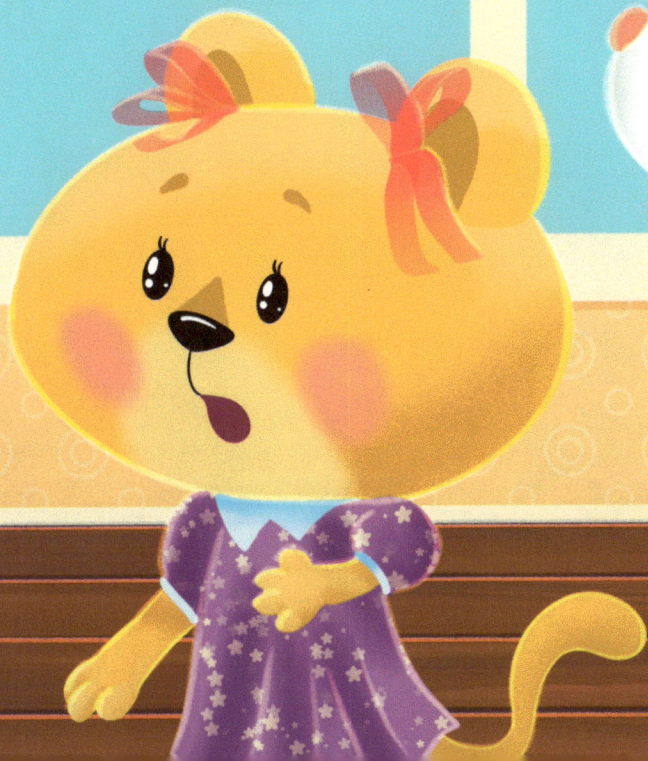

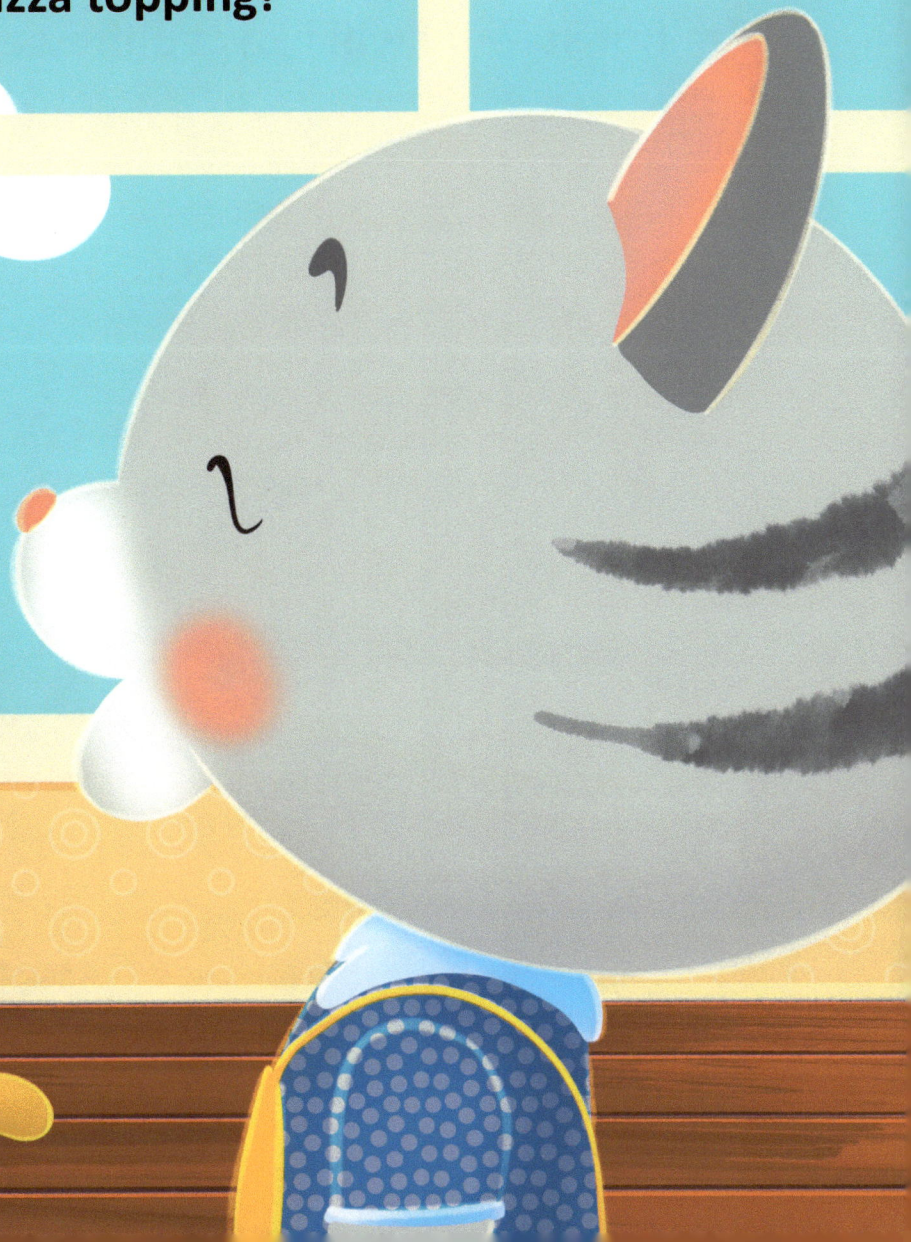

Bert asks if maybe they can try green peppers next time, and Aunt Cathy agrees!

"Tomorrow, I will get the recipe for the cauliflower tacos from my friend Davis the Duck, and we can try those!" Liza says. "I'm not sure if I will like cauliflower tacos," says Bert.

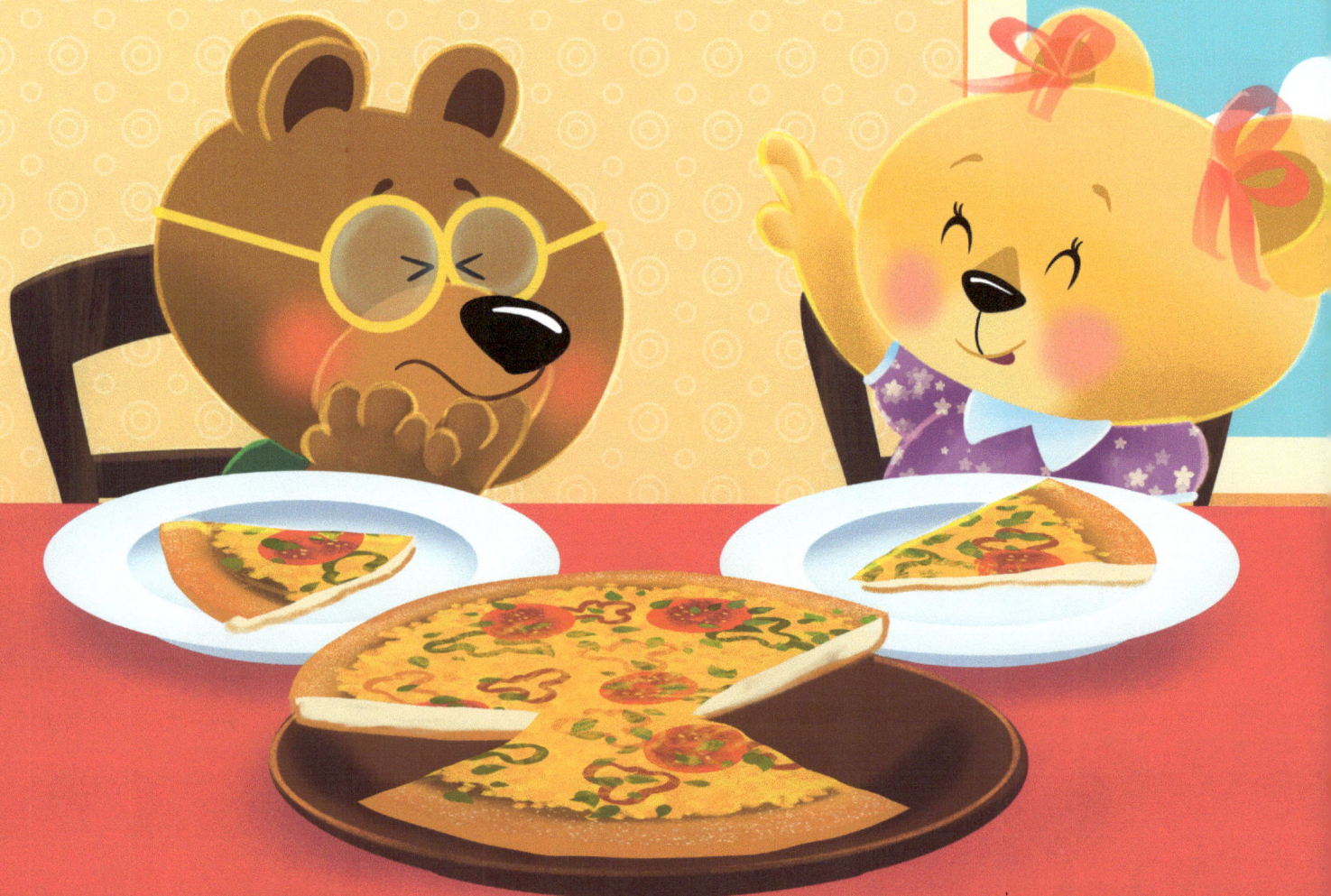

Both Aunt Cathy and Liza look at him, "BERT. . . .you won't know until you. . ."

.... and they all say together, "TRY!"

They laugh and decide to make a list of all the new vegetable pizza toppings they will try next!

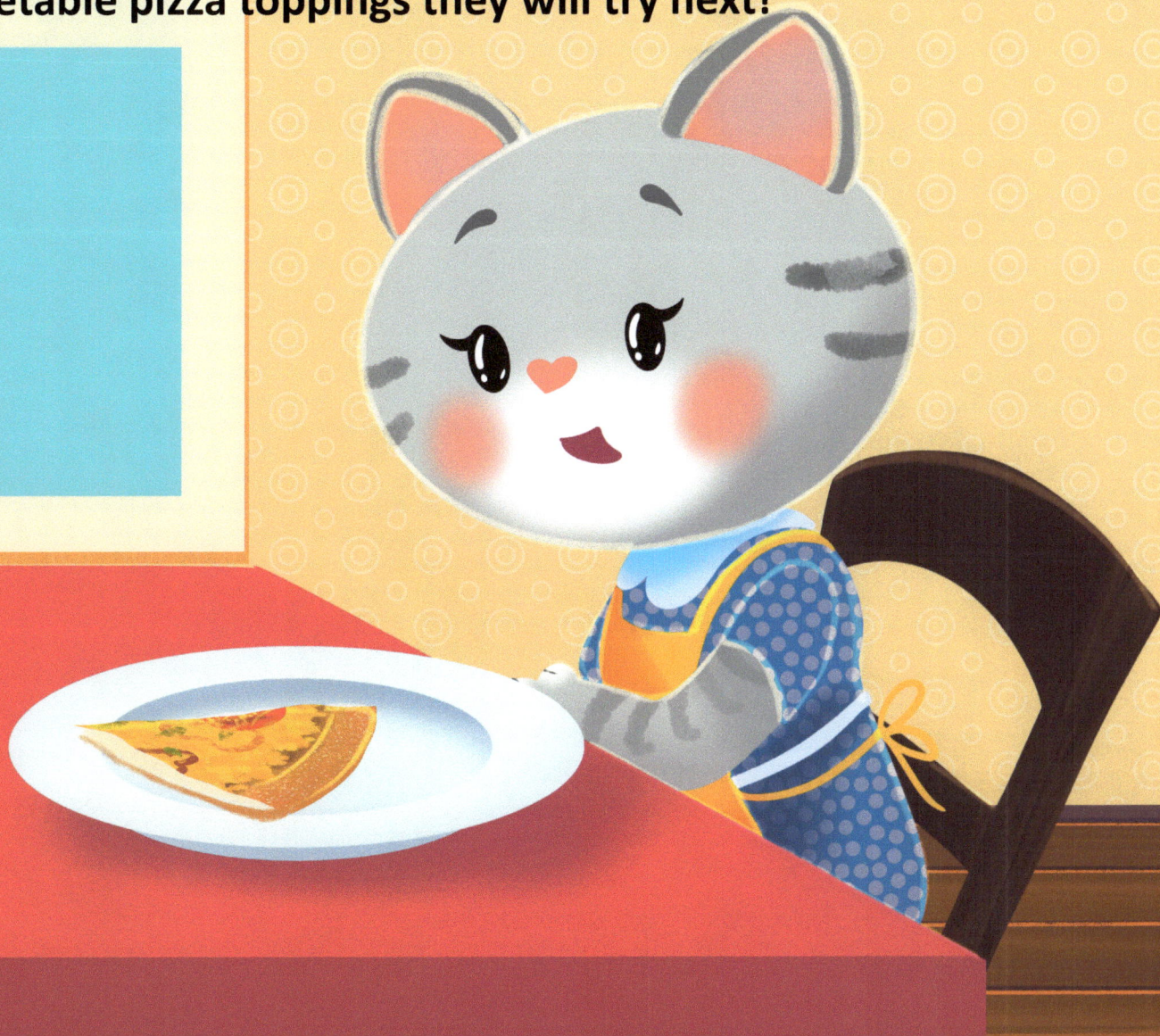

# Tips By Nurse Aimee the Alpaca on Picky Eaters!

Picky eating is common in toddlers and children. If you are a picky eater, Don't worry – it Doesn't last forever. Most picky eating is temporary! If you are unsure if you are getting enough food to grow strong and healthy, your Doctor can help check and give you advice!

## Tips for Picky Eaters (For Parents):

1. Let your kids help! Helping with shopping and preparing food helps children learn about food and get excited about creating and tasting meals. Let them pick the fruits and vegetables. Let them clean the veggies or help add ingredients or help mix ingredients.

2. Eat family meals together. Have meal times be family times. Dinner is the perfect time to catch up on what family members did that day, who they talked to, how the after-school meeting was, and how the math quiz was. Keep electronics off the table. TV off. When you can, make mealtimes something to look forward to, a time to focus on connecting as a family.

3. Be food role models! Offer the same foods to the whole family. It's okay if they don't want to try it the first time. But let them see you eating a variety of foods. Let them see you trying NEW foods. Talk about the taste, shape, color, and textures during mealtime.

## Tips for Trying New Foods (for Kids):

1. Start small! Take a tiny bite and give yourself time to get used to the taste.
2. Try new foods when you're really hungry—it might make them taste even better! Start with just one new food at a time.
3. Don't give up too quickly! It can take 10-12 tries before you start liking something new. If you don't like it one way, try it cooking it differently—steamed, baked, or sautéed might make a big difference!

## Above all – MAKE FOOD FUN!

1. Cut food into fun shapes or sizes.
2. Challenge yourself to create new snacks and new food combinations and name the dish something special, like Bert's Special Pizza!

Adapted from USDA Healthy Tips for Picky Eaters
https://wicworks.fns.usda.gov/sites/default/files/media/document/healthy-tips-for-picky-eaters-english.pdf

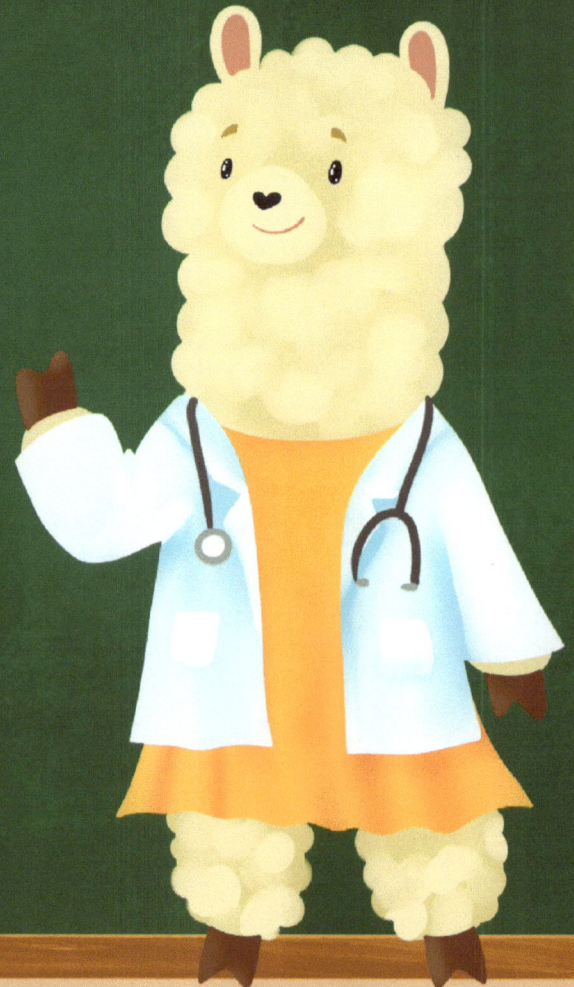

# ABout the authors

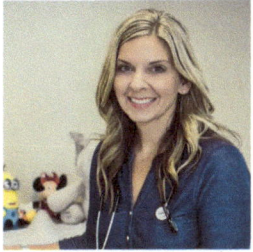

Aimee Curley, RN, MSN, earned her BS in Nursing with a degree in Nutrition from West Chester University and continued her education at Wright State University, earning her MS in Child Health and Wellness Nursing. She is the Clinical Nurse Practice Manager and Nutrition Educator at Cornerstone Pediatrics. Aimee and her husband, Tim, have two sons, Jack and Davis, and live in Chesapeake, Virginia, with their dog, Philly.

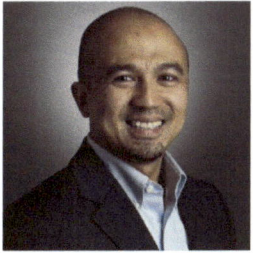

Raphael L. Aquino is the father of two amazing daughters. He is passionate about teaching children the importance of healthy habits through his nonproft, The LAB Project. The LAB Project is a 501(c)(3) nonprofit organization that aims to increase health literacy, books, and medical supplies to vulnerable and underserved children worldwide. He is a public health graduate student at Harvard T.H. Chan School of Public Health. He holds a Master's Degree in Health Care Innovation from the University of Pennsylvania, Perelman School of Medicine, and a Master's Degree in Management of Information Technology from the University of Virginia, McIntire School of Commerce.